Riddle's
Anatomy and Physiology
Applied to Health Professions

For Churchill Livingstone:

Senior commissioning editor: Sarena Wolfaard
Project manager: Derek Robertson
Design direction: Judith Wright

Riddle's
Anatomy and Physiology
Applied to Health Professions

Edited by

Jennifer Rhind BSc PhD
Faculty of Health and Life Sciences, Napier University, Edinburgh, UK

Joyce Greig BSc DipCNE CertEd RGN RCNT RNT
Faculty of Health and Life Sciences, Napier University, Edinburgh, UK

SEVENTH EDITION

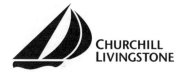

CHURCHILL
LIVINGSTONE

CHURCHILL LIVINGSTONE
An imprint of Elsevier Science Limited

First edition 1961
Second edition 1966
Third edition 1969
Fourth edition 1974
Fifth edition 1977
Sixth edition 1985
Seventh edition 2002

ISBN 0443 07031 8

British Library Cataloguing in Publication Data
A catalogue record for this book is available from the British Library

Library of Congress Cataloging in Publication Data
A catalog record for this book is available from the Library of Congress

Printed in China by RDC Group Limited

Contents

Contributors

Charlotte Chalmers BSc PhD
Lecturer, School of Life Sciences,
Napier University, Melrose, UK

12. The endocrine system
13. The reproductive system

Joyce Greig BSc DipCNE CertEd RGN RCNT RNT
Lecturer, Faculty of Health and Life Sciences,
Napier University, Edinburgh, UK

Jennifer Rhind BSc PhD
Lecturer, Faculty of Health and Life Sciences,
Napier University, Edinburgh, UK

Alison Newton MN BSc DipCNE CertEd RGN RCNT RNT
Lecturer, School of Acute and Continuing Care Nursing,
Napier University, Edinburgh, UK

9. The urinary system

Graeme Smith BA (Hons) PhD RGN
Lecturer in Nursing Studies / Research Fellow,
Department of Nursing Studies, University of Edinburgh
Edinburgh, UK

7. The digestive system

Preface

We are enormously grateful to have been given the opportunity to be associated with this book, which was first published in 1961. We have tried to remain true to J.T.E.Riddles' wish that this book should 'give the student a simple overall picture of the human body' and an 'elementary knowledge of anatomy and physiology'. It is intended for use as a basic textbook and as a stepping stone to further study.

The audience for the book encompasses all students studying anatomy and physiology at a basic level. This includes, among many others, students of nursing, complementary therapies – including aromatherapy, massage and reflexology, sports therapies, physiotherapy and occupational therapy. All chapters have been revised, particularly the skeletal system and joints, and a new chapter has been devoted to the muscles. The study questions for self-revision are retained at the end of each chapter. The book follows a systems approach, although it is appreciated that all systems work together to make up a whole that is much greater than the individual parts.

We have included text boxes with relevant, simple and interesting pathophysiology. A new feature is the marginal boxes, which are aimed at a range of student groups but which should prove of interest to all.

We are indebted to Charlotte Chalmers, Alison Newton and Graeme Smith for their contributions and we wish to thank Sarena Wolfaard and Derek Robertson for their support throughout.

2002

Jennifer Rhind,
Joyce Greig

Instructions for students

At the end of each chapter there are a variety of objective tests. These questions have been included so that you can assess your knowledge before going on to study the next system. The answers can be found on pages 187–191.

There are five different types of objective tests:

1. *Diagrams with numbered parts.* Beside each diagram is a list of lettered parts. Use this list to identify the numbered structures.

2. *Multiple choice questions.* Read the questions and from the four possible answers select the one that you think is correct.

3. *True/false questions.* These consist of a number of statements, some of which are true and some are false. Mark them 'T' for true and 'F' for false before checking with the answer list.

4. *Matching items questions.* These consist of two lists. On the left is a list of lettered items and on the right is a list of numbered items. Study the two lists and for each numbered item select the appropriate item from the lettered list.

5. *Inserting correct words.* A passage of text is printed with missing words indicated by [number]. Select the missing word represented by each number from the lettered list.

Cells, tissues, organs and systems

■ KEY POINTS

- Characteristics of life
- Organization of the body
- Cellular structure
- Transport of materials
- Cell division
- Tissues
- Body systems
- Body orientation
- Homeostasis, health and disease.

INTRODUCTION

Biology is the science that is concerned with all living systems. There are many branches of biology, including anatomy and physiology.

1. *Anatomy* (meaning 'to cut apart') is the study of the structure of a system and the relationship of one part to another; there are several branches of anatomy that will be addressed in this book, including *gross* anatomy (the study of structures that are large enough to be seen), *microscopic* anatomy (the study of the smaller structures such as cells and tissues), *regional* anatomy (the study of structures in a specified area), *systemic* anatomy (the study of body systems) and *surface* anatomy (the study of body structures in relation to the exterior surface).
2. *Physiology* is the study of the functions and processes of living systems.

Anatomy and physiology cannot be separated – form (anatomy) dictates function (physiology), and function is always related to structure. It is the relationship between the two that makes up the whole, dynamic, living system.

Before the study of anatomy and physiology commences, it is important to explore the *characteristics* of living organisms.

THE CHARACTERISTICS OF LIFE

All living things share certain characteristics. These are:

- a boundary that separates the organism from the environment
- motion
- growth
- intake of nutrients
- metabolism – the process that transforms materials taken in, and releases energy that is used by the organism
- excretion – the removal of waste products of metabolism

- responsiveness to the environment – the ability to sense and adapt to changes in the internal and external environments
- reproduction.

In order to carry out these functions, all living organisms will have basic requirements for survival. These are:

- water
- oxygen (with the exception of anaerobic organisms)
- nutrients
- appropriate external environment – temperature, atmospheric pressure.

The *cell* is the basic unit of life – all living things are comprised of cells. Even a simple, unicellular (one cell) organism has the above characteristics and needs for survival. However, the structure of the human body is more complex than that of a single-celled organism – it is comprised of many different types of cells.

THE ORGANIZATION OF THE BODY

The structure of the human body can be described at different levels of organization:

- the *cellular* level – the basic structural and functional units
- the *tissue* level – a tissue is made up of cells of the same type
- the *organ* level – an organ is a structure, made up of a variety of tissues, that has a particular function or functions
- the *system* level – a system comprises several organs that have interrelated functions that carry out a characteristic activity or activities necessary for life.

CELLULAR STRUCTURE

All animal cells, regardless of their specialized functions, share the same basic structure. Every cell has a boundary – the *cell membrane*. Inside the cell, there are small structures called *organelles* within a gelatinous substance known as *cytoplasm* (Fig. 1.1).

The cell membrane

The cell membrane (sometimes called the plasma membrane) is a very thin, flexible boundary that not only protects the contents of the cell; it also controls the passage of materials in and out of the cell. The membrane is a double layer of lipid (fat) molecules with proteins interspersed in the structure. The proteins within the structure are involved in transport across the membrane; those on the surface act as markers for identification and also as receptors for chemical signals.

Cells require nutrients, water and oxygen to survive – and these must be in solution (in a dissolved form). Products, including waste products, must also be able to pass out of the cell. Therefore, cells require a fluid environment. *Extracellular fluid* surrounds all cells of the body, and the fluid within

> Cells and tissues may be removed from the living body via various types of biopsy. The samples will be studied in the cytology laboratory, which will include a study of the cells, their origin, structure, function and pathology. This is usually carried out to determine the diagnosis.

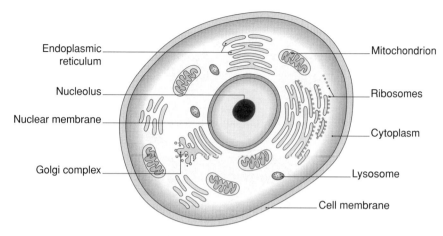

Fig. 1.1 Cellular structure (from Watson R. Essential science for nursing students: a basic introduction. London: Ballière Tindall; 1999).

the cells is known as *intracellular fluid*. The volume and composition of these must be maintained at the correct balance, so there is a constant passage of materials into the cell, and also out of the cell via the *semi-permeable* cell membrane. This means that the cell membrane will allow the passage of some molecules and can exclude others. The main transport processes across the membrane are diffusion, osmosis, filtration and active transport.

1. *Diffusion* occurs when the molecules of dissolved substances are small enough to pass through tiny pores in the membrane. Dissolved substances pass from the stronger solution to the weaker solution. This is a passive process and it does not require energy (Fig. 1.2).
2. *Osmosis* is a process where water is drawn through the membrane from the weaker solution to the stronger solution.
3. *Filtration* occurs when the pressures on each side of the membrane are not equal – the greater pressure forces fluid through the membrane.
4. *Active transport* is an energy-requiring process that moves molecules through the membrane against the concentration gradient.

There are two ways in which larger particles can enter the cell. These are both important in the body's defence – the immune system (Fig. 1.3).

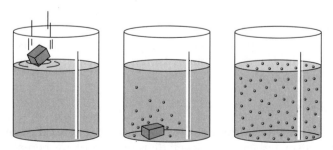

Fig. 1.2 Simple diffusion (from Salvo SG. Massage therapy: principles and practice. Philadelphia: WB Saunders; 1999).

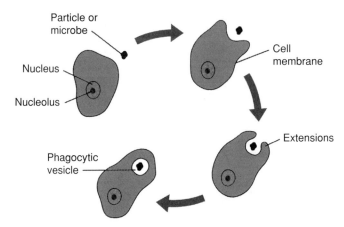

Fig. 1.3 Phagocytosis (from Salvo SG. Massage therapy: principles and practice. Philadelphia: WB Saunders; 1999).

1. *Phagocytosis* is a system where specialized cells of the immune system, such as leucocytes and macrophages in the blood, literally engulf larger foreign particles such as bacteria. Once inside the cell, the particle is digested and its remains recycled by the cell or excreted.
2. *Pinocytosis* is similar, except the engulfed substance is in liquid form.

Cytoplasm

Cytoplasm is the intracellular material. It has a gel consistency and is composed mainly of water with proteins, fats, sugars and mineral salts in solution. The fluid part is called *cytosol*, and the *cytoskeleton* gives the structure. Enzymes are present here – these are catalysts, which bring about all the biochemical reactions that are part of *metabolism*.

Metabolism is the word used to describe all of the physiological processes of the body. At the chemical level, metabolism can be considered in two distinct phases, *anabolism* and *catabolism*.

1. *Anabolism* is the process where simple molecules are built up into complex molecules such as carbohydrates, proteins, fats and nucleic acids. This requires energy. Processes such as growth, repair and reproduction are dependent on the products of anabolism.
2. *Catabolism* is the process where large, complex molecules are broken down into smaller, simple molecules – and this releases energy.

Metabolic processes are carried out by cell *organelles* – each organelle has a distinct and vital function. In every animal cell, there is a nucleus, ribosomes, endoplasmic reticulum, Golgi complex, mitochondria, lysosomes and centrosomes.

The nucleus

The nucleus is often described as the control centre of the cell, directing cellular metabolism and controlling cell division. It contains hereditary information in *genes*. DNA (deoxyribonucleic acid) is the substance that contains this inherited information, often described as the 'genetic code'.

The nucleus is spherical, and is enclosed by a nuclear membrane. Pores in this allow the passage of fairly large molecules. Within the nucleus, spherical structures – *nucleoli* – manufacture the subunits that become *ribosomes*. In cells that are not actively dividing (reproducing), *chromatin* is present. This takes the form of threads of uncoiled DNA. In cells that are reproducing, the chromatin coils and forms *chromosomes*. *Genes* are units of coded information – each gene is a segment of DNA. There are 23 pairs of chromosomes in every human cell (46 in total) except ova and spermatozoa; these contain half this number.

Ribosomes

Free ribosomes are tiny spherical structures, composed of RNA, where protein synthesis is carried out. Genetic information is transferred via RNA from the nucleus to the ribosomes; this information gives the sequence of amino acids to make proteins, which are used within the cell.

Endoplasmic reticulum

Reticulum means 'network'. Endoplasmic reticulum is an extensive system of branched tubes, channels and flattened sacs. There are two types – rough and smooth. Steroids and fatty acids are manufactured within smooth endoplasmic reticulum; this is also where fats are metabolized. Rough endoplasmic reticulum contains ribosomes – proteins are manufactured here. These are transported out of the cell for use elsewhere.

Golgi complex

The Golgi complex (sometimes called Golgi apparatus) is usually located near the nucleus. It is a stack of sacs formed by membranes, and its function is to pack and transport materials produced in the cell for use by the cell, and for release into the body.

Mitochondria

Mitochondria are large, oval organelles surrounded by an outer membrane and a folded inner membrane. Mitochondria carry out the energy-releasing functions such as respiration – the oxidation of substances to release energy.

Lysosomes

A membrane surrounds lysosomes. They contain enzymes that digest bacteria and cellular wastes. White blood cells contain large numbers of lysosomes.

Centrosome

The centrosome is a dense area near the nucleus. It contains a pair of rod-shaped structures, *centrioles*, which are important in the process of cell division.

Cell inclusions

Cells produce some substances that are stored within the cytosol – in *inclusions*. For example, glycogen, the storage carbohydrate, is stored in muscle tissue and the liver, melanin is a pigment stored in the cells of the skin and hair.

CELL DIVISION

There are two types of cell division – somatic and reproductive. Cell division is most active in fetal life and during the growing period, and also in instances where tissue needs replaced due to wear and tear or injury. The rate of growth and reproduction is controlled. If anything goes wrong with this mechanism, cell division becomes uncontrolled, and abnormal growths or tumours result.

1. *Somatic cell division* is the term used to describe the duplication of parent cells, producing identical daughter cells. This results in an increase in the number or somatic (body) cells. There are two stages to the process. *Mitosis* is the division of the nucleus, where two sets of chromosomes are divided into two separate nuclei, and *cytokinesis*, which is cytoplasmic division. The process results in two cells that are identical to the original cell.
2. *Reproductive cell division* is called *meiosis*. In this case, the chromosomes do not split, but one of each pair goes to the daughter cells. This occurs only in the male testes and female ovaries – the cells produced are known as *gametes*. The male cells (spermatozoa) and the female ova contain only 23 chromosomes, half the normal number. When the ovum and sperm fuse, a zygote containing the full complement of 46 chromosomes is formed; the child will inherit characteristics from both parents.

TISSUES

Although all cells share the same basic structure, in multicellular organisms, such as humans, many different kinds of specialized cells are found. Groups of similar cells that share the same functions are organized together to form the body *tissues*.

The study of these tissues is called histology. In the human body there are four main types of tissue, each with subdivisions. They are classed according to their structure and function:

- *epithelial* tissue – covering, lining, glandular
- *connective* tissue – protection, support, binding, storage
- *muscle* tissue – motion, movement, maintenance of posture
- *nervous* tissue – initiation and transmission of impulses, coordination.

Epithelial tissues

Epithelial tissues form the covering of the body and the lining of various organs. The cells are packed closely and arranged in sheets. *Simple* epithelium consists of one layer of cells; *stratified* epithelium is several layers thick (Fig. 1.4).

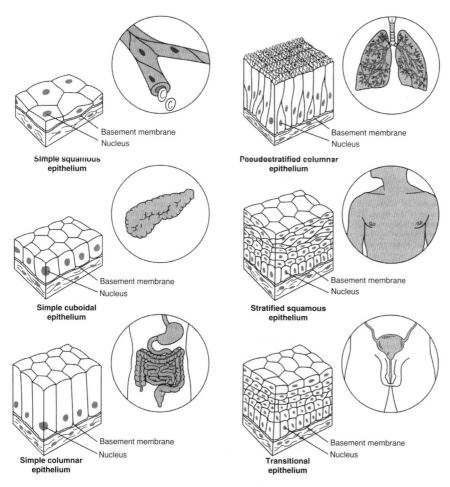

Basement membrane
Nucleus

Simple squamous
epithelium

Basement membrane
Nucleus

Pseudostratified columnar
epithelium

Basement membrane
Nucleus

Simple cuboidal
epithelium

Basement membrane
Nucleus

Stratified squamous
epithelium

Basement membrane
Nucleus

Simple columnar
epithelium

Basement membrane
Nucleus

Transitional
epithelium

Fig. 1.4 Types of epithelial tissue (from Salvo SG. Massage therapy: principles and practice. Philadelphia: WB Saunders; 1999).

Generally, simple epithelium is located in areas where there is not likely to be much 'wear and tear', and it often is specialized for absorption or filtration. Stratified epithelium is tougher – it will withstand some wear and tear. It therefore has a protective function and it will also accommodate a degree of distension and expansion of tissues. Some of the cells may be specialized for secretion.

1. *Simple squamous* epithelium consists of a single layer of thin, flattened cells. It is found in areas where wear and tear is minimal, and it is often adapted for specialized functions such as diffusion and filtration – it forms parts of the lungs, kidneys, and the blood capillaries.
2. *Simple cuboidal* epithelium consists of a single layer of cube-shaped cells that secrete and absorb substances. This type of tissue is found in the kidney tubules, ovaries, thyroid gland, pancreas and the salivary glands.

3. *Simple columnar* epithelium consists of a single layer of column-shaped cells that secrete mucus. This is commonly called mucous membrane, and it is found lining the stomach and intestines. Some of the cells are capable of absorption.
4. *Ciliated columnar* epithelium lines the respiratory passages. Here, fine hair-like projections called cilia are found on the surface of the tissue – these help to sweep the mucus and any debris away from the lungs towards the throat.
5. *Pseudostratified columnar* epithelium consists of a single layer of cells; however, it gives the appearance of being thicker due to the varying heights of the column-shaped cells. Some of the cells do not reach the surface of the tissue. This is located in parts of the respiratory tract and the male reproductive tract.
6. *Stratified squamous* epithelium consists of cells that are closely packed, and arranged in layers. The deeper layers consist of column-shaped cells and those near the surface are flattened. This tissue forms the outer layers of the skin and parts of the mouth. Its structure means that it will stand up to considerable wear and tear – the deep cells replace the superficial cells by division.
7. *Transitional* epithelium is capable of stretching under pressure. It consists of layers of cells, the shape of which varies depending on whether the tissue is relaxed or distended. When the epithelium is not under pressure, the cells appear columnar; as pressure is applied they become cuboidal then squamous shaped. Transitional epithelium is found in the bladder.
8. *Glandular* epithelium forms the glands, which are secretory structures. Some glands have ducts through which the substance is secreted, e.g. sweat glands and sebum glands in the skin. These are known as *exocrine* glands. Others are ductless, and their secretions enter the bloodstream directly. These are the *endocrine* glands and the secretions are *hormones*.

Connective tissues

Connective tissue is the most common tissue of the body. Unlike epithelial tissue, its cells are not closely packed, but are separated by a *matrix* of ground substance and thread-like fibres.

The matrix can be fluid, semi-solid, gelatinous, fibrous or rigid. The fibres are composed of collagen, elastin and reticulin:

- *collagen* is a protein that has tensile strength (it can be stretched without breaking) and flexibility
- *elastin* is a protein that is strong and elastic
- *reticulin* is a protein that can form branched networks.

The cells that comprise connective tissue include:

- *fibroblasts* – which secrete the substances that form the matrix, and produce collagen and elastin for tissue repair
- *adipocytes* – fat cells

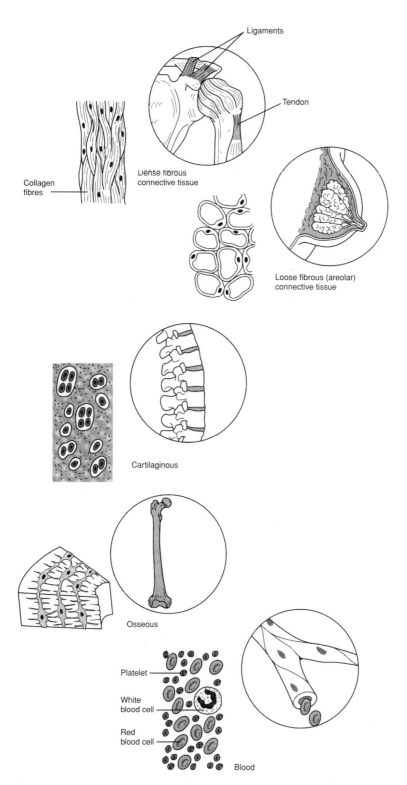

Fig. 1.5 Types of connective tissue (from Salvo SG. Massage therapy: principles and practice. Philadelphia: WB Saunders; 1999).

- *leucocytes* – white blood cells
- *mast cells* – which secrete histamine
- *plasma cells* – produce antibodies
- *macrophages* – defence mechanism.

Although connective tissue is classified into different types (Fig. 1.5), they are all interconnected, forming a protective, supportive network for the body. The types of connective tissue are:

1. *Loose connective tissue*: this is found under the skin and supporting and covering the muscles, blood vessels and nerves. It has many cells and fibres in a soft matrix. There are three types of loose connective tissue. *Areolar* tissue forms the superficial fascia of the body, attaching the skin to underlying tissues. *Adipose* tissue contains an abundance of fat cells that are specialized for storage. Adipose tissue is found in the marrow of the bones. The stored fat is an energy reserve for the body. It is also protective – it is located around the kidneys, behind the eyes and around some joints. *Reticular* tissue consists of interlaced fibres, it is supportive, and it forms the framework of some organs and binds the cells of smooth muscle.
2. *Dense connective tissue*: this has closely packed fibres, very little matrix and fewer cells. There are three types within this category. *Regular* connective tissue forms ligaments (which connect bone to bone at joints) and tendons (which connect muscle to bone). The fibres are arranged in parallel, this type of tissue can resist pulling force in one direction, but not shearing forces. *Irregular* connective tissue forms the fasciae – sheets of tissue that are supportive and protective. Fascia lines the body cavities, supports muscles and separates them into groups. Here the fibres are not regularly arranged; the tissue is able to resist forces in many directions. *Elastic* connective tissue is similar; however, its structure is not as tightly packed, its fibres are branched and yellow in colour. As the name indicates, it is elastic in nature. It is found in areas that must be able to stretch and recoil, such as the walls of the arteries, the vocal chords and in the lungs.
3. *Cartilaginous tissue*: this is very tough, protective tissue associated with the skeleton. It does not have a blood or nerve supply. Cartilaginous tissue is divided into three groups. *Hyaline cartilage* has a smooth matrix; it is bluish white in appearance, and is found covering the ends of bones involved in joint formation. *Fibrocartilage* consists of dense bundles of white fibres; it forms the discs of the spine, it forms a disc between the pubic bones (symphysis pubis) and the 'cartilage' (menisci) of the knee joints. *Elastic fibrocartilage* contains bundles of yellow fibres; it is elastic and capable of retaining shape. It forms the external ears, the nose and internally the epiglottis and auditory tubes.
4. *Bone (osseous) tissue*: this has a hard matrix and, along with cartilage, comprises the skeleton. Bone cells are called *osteocytes*, and the matrix is composed of mineral salts and collagen fibres. Bone tissue may be *compact* (dense) or *cancellous* (spongy).

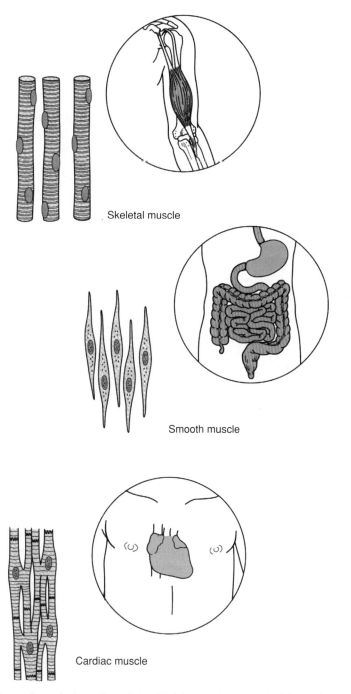

Skeletal muscle

Smooth muscle

Cardiac muscle

Fig. 1.6 Types of muscle tissue (from Salvo SG. Massage therapy: principles and practice. Philadelphia: WB Saunders; 1999).

5. *Blood (vascular or haemopoietic) tissue*: this has a liquid matrix known as *plasma*. The cells suspended in the plasma are *erythrocytes* (red blood cells), *leucocytes* (white blood cells) and also *thrombocytes* or *platelets*.

Muscle tissue

Muscle tissue is capable of contraction and thus provides motion and movement. There is little intercellular substance and the cells (known as *muscle fibres*) are closely packed. There are three types of muscle tissue – *skeletal*, *smooth* and *cardiac* (Fig. 1.6).

1. *Skeletal muscle tissue* forms the muscles that are responsible for the movement of the skeleton and the maintenance of posture. It is also known as *striated* muscle, as it has a striped appearance under the microscope, or *voluntary* muscle, because it is under conscious control. Skeletal muscle cells are elongated and striated with light and dark bands. They contain many nuclei at the periphery of each cell.
2. *Smooth muscle tissue* forms the walls of the internal organs, the viscera. It is also called involuntary muscle because it is not under conscious control. The cells are elongated and spindle-shaped, but not striated. Each contains one nucleus.
3. *Cardiac muscle tissue* is the muscle tissue of the heart wall. It is not located anywhere else in the body and it is not under conscious control. Striations are apparent under the microscope. The cells are shaped like the letters 'Y' and 'H'; this allows them to fit closely together and form the spherical shape of the heart.

Nervous tissue

This is the tissue that forms the brain, the spinal cord and the nerves. It coordinates all body activities. The cells are called *neurons*; these can initiate, transmit and interpret signals (impulses). Connective tissue cells called *neuroglia* support, nourish and protect neurons.

BODY SYSTEMS

Tissues are organized to form *organs*. A *system* is a collection of organs that work together to fulfil a particular function or functions. Each system carries out one or more of the vital functions of the body, but none of the systems can work independently. The body systems, their component organs and functions are summarized in Table 1.1.

BODY ORIENTATION

The anatomical parts of the body

The body may be divided into four parts – the *head and neck*, the *trunk*, the *upper limbs* and the *lower limbs*. The organs and structures are contained within enclosed *cavities*. The largest body cavities (Fig. 1.7) are:

- The *cranial cavity*, which contains the brain.
- The *thoracic cavity* – the uppermost cavity of the trunk; it contains the lungs, the heart, large blood vessels and the oesophagus.
- The *abdominal cavity*, which is the largest cavity in the trunk. The abdominal organs are the stomach, the intestines, the liver, the pancreas,

Table 1.1 Overview of the body systems

System	Organs	Functions
Skeletal	The bones of the axial and appendicular skeleton	Framework, support and protection, production of blood cells, storage of minerals
Muscular	Skeletal, smooth and cardiac muscle	Motion and movement
Integumentary	Skin, hair, nails, exocrine glands	Sensation, protection, excretion, temperature regulation, reservoir for blood, synthesis of vitamin D
Cardiovascular (circulatory)	Heart, blood vessels, blood	Transport of nutrients, gases (oxygen) and hormones to the body cells
Lymphatic/immune	Bone, lymph vessels, lymph nodes, spleen, thymus, lymphoid tissue	Defence, return of extracellular fluid to the blood, formation of white blood cells
Respiratory	Nose, pharynx, larynx, bronchi, bronchioles, lungs	Exchange of oxygen and carbon dioxide
Digestive	Mouth, pharynx, oesophagus, stomach, intestines, bowel; accessory organs are the salivary glands, pancreas, liver, gall bladder	Ingestion, digestion and absorption of food and elimination of the residue
Urinary	Kidneys, ureters, urinary bladder, urethra	Excretion of waste materials from the body
Nervous	Brain, spinal cord and nerves. Also the special sense organs – hearing, sight and smell	Regulation and coordination of all the body functions and interaction with the external environment, states of consciousness. Maintenance of homeostasis
Endocrine	Glands – pituitary, thyroid, parathyroid, adrenal, pancreas, testes, ovaries, thymus, pineal	Regulation and coordination of body functions via hormones
Reproductive	Male – testes, penis. Female – ovaries, uterus, vagina, mammary glands	Male – production of sperm. Female – production of ova, nurtures embryo

the spleen and the kidneys. The abdominal cavity is divided into nine regions so that the positions of these organs can be identified (Fig. 1.8).

- The *pelvic cavity*, which contains the reproductive organs, the ureters and bladder, and the lower part of the bowel.

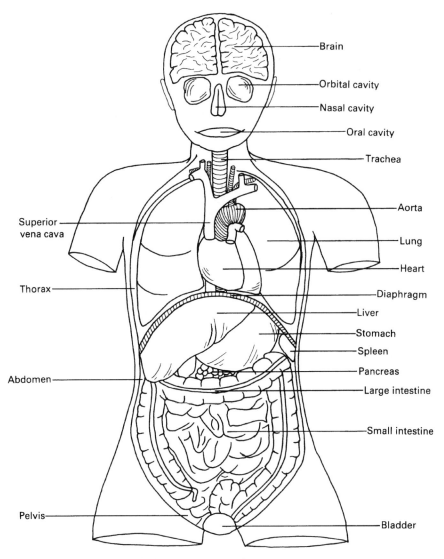

Fig. 1.7 Head, neck and trunk, showing organs and cavities.

Anatomical terminology

Specific terminology is used to describe the parts of the body and their orientation. All of these terms are used in relation to the *anatomical position*:

- the *anatomical position* – the body is erect, with the arms at the sides, palms facing forwards and thumbs outward, and the toes pointing forwards
- the *midline of the body* - is an imaginary vertical line running from the top of the head down the trunk, dividing the body into two sides.

The following terms are commonly used:

- *anterior* or *ventral* – in front of, or towards the front

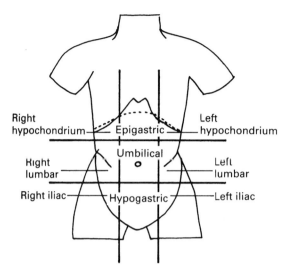

Fig. 1.8 Regions of the abdomen.

- *posterior* or *dorsal* – behind, towards the back or rear
- *proximal* – point closer to the trunk or point of origin
- *distal* – point situated away from the trunk, or midline, or point of origin
- *medial* – nearer to the midline
- *lateral* – away from the midline, to the outer side
- *superior* – higher than, or above
- *inferior* – lower than, below
- *internal* – an inner surface, or the inner part of the body
- *external* – the outer surface of the body
- *palmar* – the anterior aspect of the hand (the palm)
- *plantar* – the sole of the foot.

HOMEOSTASIS, HEALTH AND DISEASE

Homeostasis

Our physiological processes allow us to function in a balanced state – the cells that make up the tissues and organs must be maintained in their optimum environment. Factors such as temperature, pressure and chemical composition of our body fluids must be kept within defined parameters. The name given to this constant state is *homeostasis*, and this is necessary for good health.

All of the body systems contribute to maintaining homeostasis. However, the nervous system and endocrine systems are largely responsible for the regulation and coordination of our internal environment, and responses to changes in the external environment. Good health depends largely on how well we can adapt to changes and maintain a balance.

Feedback mechanisms

This dynamic control system consists of feedback mechanisms. These feedback mechanisms (feedback loops) have the following features:

- *a detector* – a sensor that will respond to nervous impulses or chemical changes
- *a control centre* – where the responses are analysed and integrated, and the limits for response are set
- an *effector* – a mechanism that responds to restore balance.

Most feedback loops are *negative feedback* mechanisms, because the response from the effector negates the effects of whatever stimulated the detector in the first instance. *Positive feedback* mechanisms are less common; in these cases the response from the effector will further stimulate the detector, so that a disturbed state continues for a time. This only serves a purpose in a few circumstances, such as maintaining contractions during labour.

Homeostatic imbalance

If the control mechanisms fail to provide balance in the body's internal environment, and homeostasis is not achieved, dysfunction of the cells, tissues, organs and body systems will result.

Many complementary therapies are believed to either support or stimulate homeostasis, thus helping the body to maintain or regain a state of balance.

Disease is the abnormal functioning of the body that affects well being, and may give rise to symptoms of a specific illness. *Pathology* is the name given to the study of disease, and how it affects the body structure and function. *Pathophysiology* is the study of the physiological processes of disease.

In a healthy state, we are able to adapt to changes, and our homeostatic mechanisms will restore the essential balance. Disease occurs when the body cannot adapt.

Many factors can disturb homeostasis, including exposure to toxic substances, radiation, injury, extremes of temperature, malnutrition and exposure to infections. Also, some diseases will have effects that further contribute to the disturbance.

However, genetic factors (what we inherit) will play a role in the individual's regulatory mechanisms, homeostasis is affected by the natural ageing process, and an excess of stress can place heavy demands on the body's ability to maintain homeostasis (Box 1.1). In addition, some lifestyle habits can also cause homeostatic imbalance, for example, poor diet, smoking, lack of exercise, excessive use of alcohol, drugs.

■ BOX 1.1 Stress and illness

The causes of stress may be a combination of physical, environmental, mental, emotional or spiritual factors, and the individual will invariably be affected on several levels. Many illnesses are thought to be stress related, although often the exact nature of the link is not understood. *Psychophysiology* (the study of the relationship between the mind and physiology) and *psychoneuroimmunology* (the mind and its links with the nervous and immune systems) are two relatively new disciplines, which seek to explore and quantify the mind–body connection.

CELLS, TISSUES, ORGANS AND SYSTEMS QUESTIONS

Diagrams—Questions 1–20

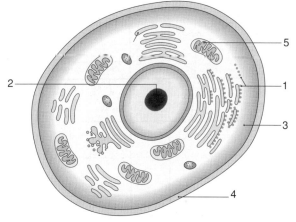

1–5. A cell

A. Cell membrane
B. Nucleolus
C. Ribosomes
D. Mitochondrion
E. Cytoplasm

1
2
3
4
5

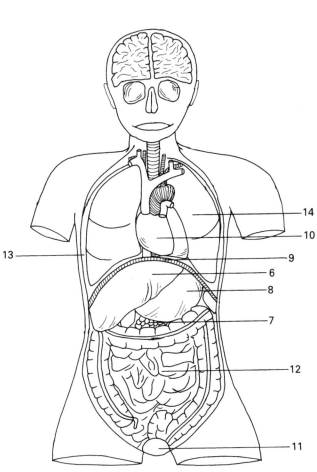

6–14. Head, neck and trunk

A. Diaphragm
B. Bladder
C. Heart
D. Intestine
E. Liver
F. Lungs
G. Pancreas
H. Stomach
I. Thorax

6
7
8
9
10
11
12
13
14

15–20. Regions of the abdomen

A. Hypogastric region
B. Epigastric region
C. Left hypochondrium region
D. Left iliac region
E. Left lumbar region
F. Umbilical region

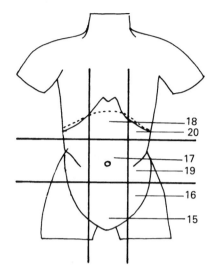

15
16
17
18
19
20

Questions 21–35 are of the multiple choice type

21. Which one of the following parts of a cell contains the genes?   21
A. Lysosome
B. Chromosome
C. Endoplasmic reticulum
D. Mitochondrion.

22. Zygote is the name given to: 22
A. the female egg cell
B. the fertilized ovum
C. the male sex cell
D. all sex cells.

23. Osmosis occurs when: 23
A. increased pressure forces a solution through a membrane
B. a concentrated solution draws fluid from a weak solution
C. solids pass across a semi-permeable membrane
D. water passes across a permeable membrane.

24. The number of chromosomes in each ordinary human cell is: 24
A. 22
B. 23
C. 44
D. 46.

25. The number of chromosomes in a gamete is: 25
A. 22
B. 23
C. 44
D. 46.

26. Tissues: 26
A. are all soft in consistency
B. consist of a number of different cells
C. consist of a number of similar cells
D. have only one function.

27. Epithelium is the tissue which forms: 27
A. coverings for organs
B. linings for organs
C. walls of organs
D. tendons and ligaments.

28. Which one of the following epithelial tissues forms the outer part of the skin?   28
A. Ciliated
B. Cuboid
C. Stratified
D. Transitional.

29. Which one of the following is not a connective tissue?   29
A. Blood
B. Bone
C. Cartilage
D. Muscle.

30. Tendons: 30
A. are made of areolar tissue
B. are made of white fibro-cartilage
C. join muscle to bone
D. join bone to bone.

31. Hyaline cartilage: 31
A. has a soft matrix
B. contains calcium
C. forms part of the structure of a bone
D. forms ligaments.

32. Skeletal muscle tissue cells are: 32
A. branched
B. plain
C. striped
D. striped and branched.

33. Which one of the following organs is part of the circulatory system?   33
A. Pancreas
B. Spleen
C. Pharynx
D. Lungs.

34. Which one of the following organs does not excrete waste?   34
A. Pancreas
B. Kidneys
C. Lungs
D. Skin.

35. A hormone is: 35
A. part of a cell
B. a chemical product of a gland
C. part of the nervous system
D. a gland with a duct.

The skeletal system

KEY POINTS

- Introduction
- The functions of the skeleton
- Classification of bones
- The structure of bones
- The growth and development of bone
- Bony landmarks

- The bones of the axial skeleton
- The bones of the thorax
- The bones of the appendicular skeleton
- Common disorders and implications for bodywork and nursing.

The study of the bones that comprise the skeleton is important for all bodywork and movement therapists. For example, knowledge of bony landmarks is required for the study of surface anatomy; bodywork students must learn the *origins* and *insertions* of muscles (attachments to bones at specific points). The reflexologist requires a detailed knowledge of the bones of the hands and feet.

INTRODUCTION

The skeletal system consists of the bones, joints and their connective tissue components that give the body its framework.

FUNCTIONS OF THE SKELETON

The functions of the skeleton are to provide:

- support – the skeletal framework supports the soft tissues and the body weight
- protection – for delicate internal organs such as the brain, spinal cord, bladder, etc.
- attachment – for ligaments and tendons
- leverage – allows movement via the attached muscles.

In addition, the tissues of the skeletal system have important roles to play in the physiological processes of the body:

- storage of fats (for use as an energy source) and minerals such as calcium and phosphorus
- production of red blood cells in red bone marrow; this function is known as *haemopoesis*.

CLASSIFICATION OF BONES

The bones are made up of several different tissues and have different shapes. The location and shape of a bone will determine its function within the skeleton. However, each bone belongs to only one of four categories: long, short, flat and irregular.

Long bones

The long bones (Fig. 2.1) are found in the limbs, and because of their shape and method of attachment to each other they allow movement. A long bone is characterized by a tubular shaft (the *diaphysis*) with a central cavity (the *medullary canal*) and one or two rounded extremities (the *epiphysis*).

Short bones

Short bones do not have a uniform shape. They are often found collected together in groups – for example, at the wrists and ankles, where they form strong units that can support the weight of the body. Sometimes these are classed as *cube-shaped* bones. *Sesamoid* bones are often grouped in this category. These are round bones, which are found embedded in tendons and joint capsules – the patella (kneecap) is an example. Smaller sesamoid bones are located in the hands and feet.

Flat bones

As the name indicates, these bones are flat in form (Fig. 2.2). They form the walls of the major body cavities and protect their contents. For example, the bones of the skull, thorax and pelvis are flat bones.

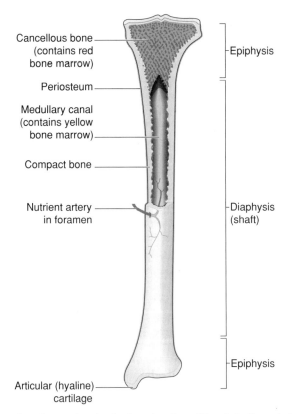

Fig. 2.1 A mature long bone – longitudinal section (from Waugh A, Grant A. Ross and Wilson Anatomy and physiology in health and illness. 9th edn. Edinburgh: Churchill Livingstone; 2001).

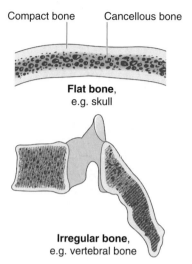

Compact bone   Cancellous bone

Flat bone,
e.g. skull

Irregular bone,
e.g. vertebral bone

Fig. 2.2 Flat and irregular bones (from Waugh A, Grant A. Ross and Wilson Anatomy and physiology in health and illness. 9th edn. Edinburgh: Churchill Livingstone; 2001).

Irregular bones

Irregular bones generally have complex shapes (Fig. 2.2). The vertebrae and the facial bones are examples of irregular bones.

THE STRUCTURE OF BONES

All bones are made of the same types of tissue, regardless of their form or function. The tissues that form the bones are all classed as *connective tissue*:

- bone tissue, or *osseous* tissue
- fibrous tissue
- hyaline cartilage
- adipose tissue.

The common perception is that bones are somewhat lifeless and static; however, bones are in fact dynamic structures. Bone is constantly changing and remodelling to meet the body's needs.

Bone is a relatively hard material that consists of 25% water and 75% solids. Bone cells, an organic matrix, and calcium and phosphorus mineral salts are the main constituents of the solid portion.

Bone tissue

There are two types of bone tissue, light *cancellous* bone and dense *compact* bone (Fig. 2.3).

1. *Cancellous* bone tissue has a spongy appearance; it is full of little spaces that are surrounded by thin plates of bone. This makes the structure lighter in weight than compact bone. The thin plates of bone that form a mesh-like structure are known as *trabeculae*. In some bones, the trabecular spaces are filled with red bone marrow. Cancellous bone is located at

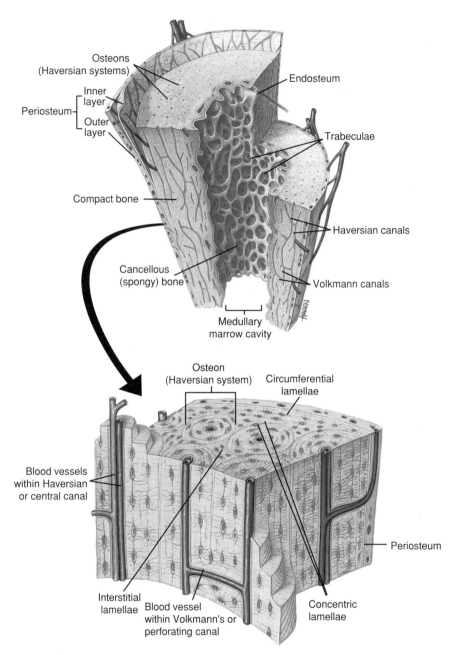

Fig. 2.3 Structure of cancellous and compact bone. (A) Longitudinal section of a long bone, showing both cancellous and compact bone. (B) Magnified view of compact bone. (From Fritz S, Paholsky KM, Grosenbach MJ. Mosby's basic science for soft tissue and movement therapies. St Louis: Mosby; 1998.)

the extremities of long bones, the centre of short bones and sandwiched between the compact plates of flat bones.

2. *Compact* bone tissue forms a hard shell, which varies in thickness, and gives the bone strength. It protects cancellous bone, and provides the firm framework of the skeleton. Although solid in appearance in com-

parison with cancellous bone tissue, it too is composed of a mesh-like structure. However, the tiny plates of bone are much closer together and are arranged in a concentric manner. These are known as *lammellae*. Bone cells (*osteophytes*) are located in the spaces between the plates, and in rings around central canals. Central *Haversian canals* are found in compact bone. These are tiny vascular canals that run longitudinally through the bone – a route for nerves and blood vessels. Haversian canals are connected by *Volkmann's canals*.

Fibrous tissue

A sheath of fibrous tissue adheres to all the surfaces of each bone, except where joints are formed. This is the *periosteum* – a protective covering that also penetrates the bone. Periosteum has important functions:

1. It is supplied with blood and lymph vessels, and therefore plays an important role in the nourishment of bone tissue. If a bone specimen is examined, small 'scratches' can be observed on the shaft. These are the openings through which blood vessels of the periosteum enter the bone.
2. It is supplied with nerves – thus pain is experienced if bone tissue is damaged or traumatized.
3. It serves as a point of attachment for tendons and ligaments.
4. The inner part of the periosteum contains bone cells known as *osteoblasts* – bone-forming cells that are important in growth or repair of bone.

A thinner membrane of fibrous tissue is found lining the medullary canal. This is the *endosteum*. Bone cells that are important in growth and repair are associated with this membrane.

Hyaline cartilage

Hyaline (or *articular*) cartilage is a smooth, slippery, translucent, blue-white connective tissue that is located at the extremities of long bones, and wherever there is a moveable joint. It is *avascular* (it does not have a blood supply) and is not supplied with nerves, thus it is insensitive. Hyaline cartilage allows the bones to glide freely on one another.

Adipose tissue

Two types of adipose tissue are involved in bone structure – *red* and *yellow bone marrow*.

1. *Red bone marrow* is the fatty tissue found in the spaces in cancellous bone. This tissue has a very important function, as it is here that the blood cells are developed and matured before they are released into the bloodstream. Red bone marrow is located at the extremities of long bones and in the central parts of bones of the thorax and pelvis.
2. *Yellow bone marrow* is mainly fat, found in medullary cavities. This store of fat is an energy source, and is released as required by the body.

Infants up to the age of 5 years have red bone marrow in the medullary canals of their long bones. This is gradually replaced by yellow bone marrow, containing more fat cells and fewer blood cells.

THE GROWTH AND DEVELOPMENT OF BONE

The growth and development of bone is influenced by:

- hormones – including *growth hormone*, and the *sex hormones* during puberty
- dietary factors – including the amount of *calcium phosphate* (found in dairy products and green vegetables) and *vitamin D* (found in animal fats, cod liver oil) in the diet (vitamin D is manufactured in the skin when exposed to the ultraviolet rays of sunlight; it has many functions, including the metabolism of calcium).

The fetal skeleton

The fetal skeleton is made of tough, flexible cartilage, created by *chondroblasts* (cartilage-forming cells). Bone-forming cells, *osteoblasts*, transform the cartilage structure into bone tissue.

Osteoblasts take calcium from the blood supply and incorporate it into small plates in the cartilage. This normally starts in the middle of the shaft of a long bone at the *primary centre of ossification* (Fig. 2.4). From this centre, calcium is laid down in both directions, forming the shaft of the bone. The shaft (*diaphysis*) becomes longer. The laying down of calcium, which, in the presence of vitamin D, has been absorbed from food and carried in the bloodstream to the fetus, gradually hardens the relatively flexible fetal skeleton.

Babies and children

After birth, calcification continues, and the bones continue to harden. The process is called *ossification* (or *osteogenesis*). *Secondary centres* of ossification develop at the extremities of bones (Fig. 2.4). The ossified extremities are called the epiphyses. Between the diaphysis and the epiphysis is a plate of cartilage, called the epiphyseal cartilage, which is the growth area of the bone (Fig. 2.4). It remains until growth is complete, and can be seen on an X-ray plate as a space between the shaft and the extremity.

Puberty

Ossification is not completed until the early twenties. There is often a 'growth spurt' at puberty and in the teens, due to the influence of the sex hormones. Boys are generally taller and have denser bones due to the presence of testosterone; the influence of oestrogen prevents the further growth of long bone. During the growth phase the bones also become thicker.

■ **BOX 2.1 Rickets**

Rickets is a childhood nutritional disorder. Vitamin D deficiency prevents the absorption of calcium and phosphorus, so that these minerals cannot be laid down in the bones. The bones become soft and deformed, sometimes resulting in 'knock knees' or 'bow legs'. Rickets is now rare in the West.

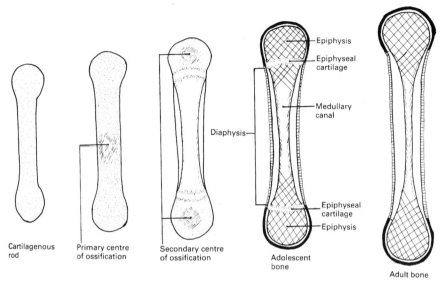

Fig. 2.4 Development of a long bone.

Adult and ageing skeleton

Other cells are important during growth and subsequent development. *Osteoclasts* are cells that break down bone tissue, either to maintain homeostasis or to repair damage. *Osteocytes* are mature osteoblasts (bone forming-cells), which are incorporated into the bone matrix.

In adults, when ossification is complete, the skeleton is more rigid. It is also more brittle, containing more minerals, more bone cells than cartilage and fewer blood vessels. Thus, fractures take longer to heal.

As ageing progresses, loss of calcium can become a problem, especially in females.

A client with brittle, soft or fragile bones must not be subjected to any treatment that involves compressive force or joint movement (unless under medical supervision). In such circumstances, any massage must be light and superficial.

■ BOX 2.2 Growing pains

General 'growing pains' can occur in adolescents during a growth 'spurt'. If the bone is growing faster than the surrounding muscles, the tendons will pull on their points of attachment to the sensitive periosteum, causing pain.

■ BOX 2.3 Osteoporosis

Osteoporosis is a bone demineralization disorder. It is most common in post-menopausal women, due to hormonal influences, but can also be caused by faulty diet, or absorption of nutrients and minerals. Inactivity and smoking are contributing factors. In osteoporosis, minerals such as calcium are lacking and the bone-forming process is slower, so that the bones become fragile and prone to fracture.

Fractures

The fractured limb and the plaster must be observed continually for:

- swelling
- irritation
- leakage from wounds
- cracks in the plaster
- a foul smell which may indicate the presence of infection
- increasing levels of pain.

Always report any of the above.

Force, if severe enough, can *fracture* (break) bones. Fractures are not common in young children, but in time the bones become progressively harder, and in old age, they may be quite brittle – even a trivial injury can result in a fracture. The signs and symptoms may include swelling, loss of function, pain, and abnormal movement or appearance. A grating sound or sensation may be heard or felt – this is *crepitus*.

First aid measures should include the immobilization of the affected part, and seeking medical aid as quickly as possible.

The more common fractures are:

- simple (closed) fractures – where the broken bone does not protrude through the skin
- open (compound) fractures – where a broken bone breaks through the soft tissue and protrudes through the skin
- stress fractures – small cracks in the bone, due to repeated mechanical stress on the structure.

Other types of fracture include:

- comminuted fracture – where there are more than one fractures of a bone, resulting in several fragments
- compression fracture – where a bone is squeezed or crushed
- greenstick fracture – where a bone snaps on one side and then tears lengthwise, resembling a split in a twig; this is a more common type of fracture in children, and it heals fairly quickly.

Healing

Blood fills the area surrounding the fracture and, within 2 or 3 days, a *fracture haematoma* (blood clot) forms. Gradually, granulation tissue replaces the haematoma, and osteoblasts and chondroblasts begin to form new bone and cartilage tissue. After about a week, a *procallus* (a temporary bony union) is formed. A rigid, bony *callus* eventually replaces this.

Generally, depending on type and severity, fractures will take about 6 weeks to heal. Immobilization is often necessary to allow the healing process to progress to a satisfactory outcome. Any associated soft-tissue damage may also require medical treatment.

FEATURES OF BONES

The shapes of bones are related to their functions within the skeleton. Bony features such as depressions, openings and various protuberances are regions where nerves and vessels enter and leave, or muscles attach. The most common terms relating to these bony landmarks are given in Table 2.1.

THE BONES OF THE SKELETON

The skeleton (Fig. 2.5) is usually described in two divisions, the *axial* skeleton and the *appendicular* skeleton. The axial skeleton comprises the bones

Table 2.1 Bony landmarks

Bony feature	Definition
Fissure	A groove between two bones
Foramen	An opening in a bone, allows passage of nerves, blood vessels
Fossa	A depression in the surface of a bone, or at the end of a bone
Groove	A narrow depression that accommodates blood vessels, nerves, tendons
Notch	An indentation in a bone
Sinus	An air cavity within a bone
Crest	A ridge on a bone, for muscle attachment
Condyle	A rounded projection at the end of a bone (joint formation)
Epicondyle	A projection superior to a condyle
Process	A prominent bony projection
Spinous process	A slender bony projection
Head	A rounded projection superior to the neck of a bone
Trochanter	A large bony process (only found on the femur)
Tubercle	A small, rounded process
Tuberosity	A large, rounded process
Trochlea	A pulley-shaped structure
Line	A very small ridge
Facet	A smooth, flat surface

of the head and trunk – it is the central support, or axis, of the body. The appendicular skeleton comprises the limbs of the body and is connected to the axial skeleton by the shoulder girdle and pelvis.

THE SPINAL OR VERTEBRAL COLUMN

Humans are described as *vertebrates* – this term means that a spine, or vertebral column, is an important distinguishing feature of our anatomy.

- The spine is a series of small, irregular bones (*vertebrae*) that are attached to each other in such a way that the spine can carry out its functions – protection of the spinal cord, central support for the body and mobility.

Regions

Thirty-three vertebrae comprise the human vertebral column. The vertebrae are grouped into five regions:

- cervical – the neck
- thoracic – the back
- lumbar – the lower back
- sacral – the pelvis
- coccygeal – the 'tail'.

Curves

If the spine is viewed from the side it will be seen that it is not straight but forms four curves. These curves are not all present at birth, but develop gradually. The development of the curves of the spine is shown in Figure 2.6.

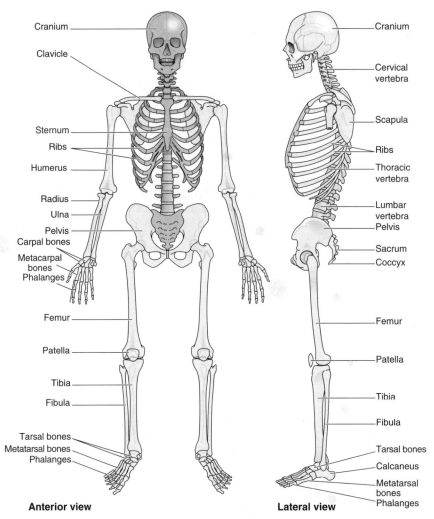

Fig. 2.5 The skeleton – anterior and lateral views (from Waugh A, Grant A. Ross and Wilson Anatomy and physiology in health and illness. 9th edn. Edinburgh: Churchill Livingstone; 2001).

The curves of the spine are the:

- cervical curve, which is convex to the anterior
- thoracic curve, which is concave to the anterior
- lumbar curve, which is convex to the anterior
- sacral curve, which is concave to the anterior.

■ **BOX 2.4 Abnormal spinal curves**

Abnormal curves of the spine are fairly common. These may be due to postural deficiencies, or may be congenital. *Scoliosis* is a lateral bending of the vertebral column – usually affecting the thoracic region. *Kyphosis* is an exaggerated thoracic curve, often described as 'round shoulders'. *Lordosis* is an exaggerated lumbar curve.

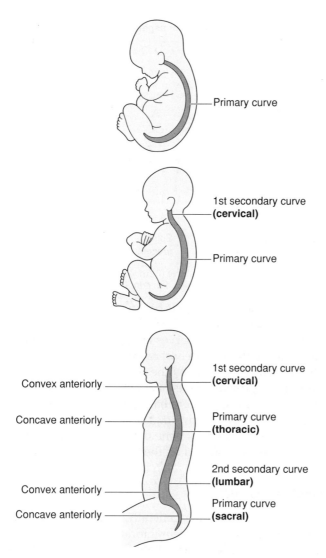

Primary curve

1st secondary curve
(cervical)

Primary curve

1st secondary curve
(cervical)

Convex anteriorly

Concave anteriorly

Primary curve
(thoracic)

2nd secondary curve
(lumbar)

Convex anteriorly

Primary curve
(sacral)

Concave anteriorly

Fig. 2.6 Diagram showing the order of development of the curves of the spine (from Waugh A, Grant A. Ross and Wilson Anatomy and physiology in health and illness. 9th edn. Edinburgh: Churchill Livingstone; 2001).

These curves increase the strength of the spine, they help maintain balance in an upright position, they absorb shock when walking and also help protect the column from damage.

Vertebrae

The 24 separate, moveable vertebrae are found in the *cervical, thoracic* and *lumbar* regions. They are similar in structure (Figs 2.7 and 2.8), with a few exceptions.

Each vertebra has the following features:

1. A box shaped *body* lies towards the front and bears the weight.

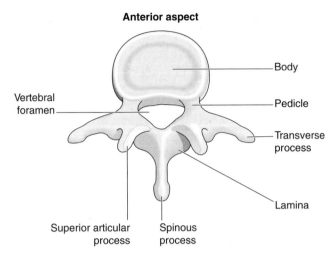

Fig. 2.7 A typical vertebra, viewed from above (from Waugh A, Grant A. Ross and Wilson Anatomy and physiology in health and illness. 9th edn. Edinburgh: Churchill Livingstone; 2001).

2. A *vertebral* (or *neural*) *arch* projects backwards, enclosing an opening known as the *vertebral foramen*. This is part of the *vertebral canal*. The *spinal cord*, which carries the nerves from the brain to all parts of the body, passes through the vertebral canal.
3. The arch is joined to the body by the *pedicles*.
4. Three projections provide points of attachment for muscles that move the spinal column. Each vertebra has a prominent *spinous process* (these can be easily palpated), and two *transverse processes*.
5. The *laminae* are flat sections of bone that form the back of the arch.
6. *Articulating processes* are found on the laminae – these form little joints that allow each vertebra to move on its neighbour.

The cervical vertebrae

There are seven cervical vertebrae; generally, they are smaller than the others and have three openings – the vertebral foramen, and two smaller openings in the transverse processes, which allow passage of blood vessels to the brain. The first two cervical vertebrae – the *atlas* and the *axis* – are not typical.

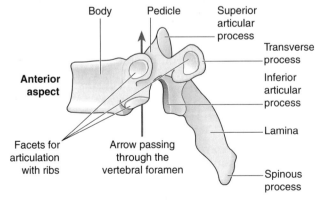

Fig. 2.8 A typical vertebra, viewed from the side (from Waugh A, Grant A. Ross and Wilson Anatomy and physiology in health and illness. 9th edn. Edinburgh: Churchill Livingstone; 2001).

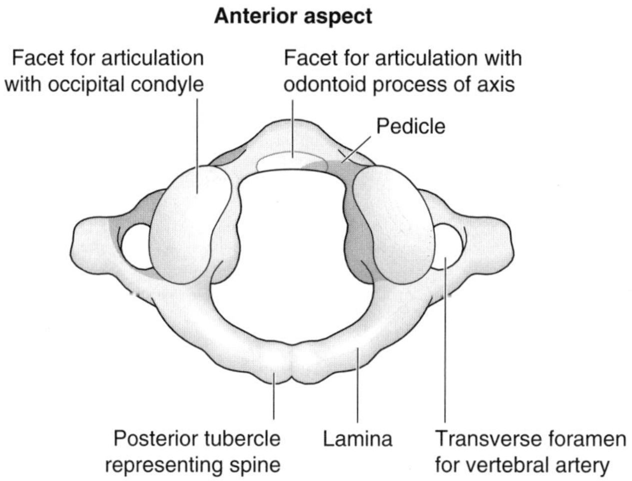

Anterior aspect

Facet for articulation with occipital condyle

Facet for articulation with odontoid process of axis

Pedicle

Posterior tubercle representing spine

Lamina

Transverse foramen for vertebral artery

Fig. 2.9 The atlas viewed from above (from Waugh A, Grant A. Ross and Wilson Anatomy and physiology in health and illness. 9th edn. Edinburgh: Churchill Livingstone; 2001).

The *atlas* (Fig. 2.9) is a ring of bone with no body and two short transverse processes. It has a large foramen for the beginning of the spinal cord. There are two facets that provide for articulation with the skull, allowing nodding movements of the head.

The *atlas* is the second cervical vertebra. It has a tooth-like process, called the *odontoid process* (or *dens*), which projects upward from the body. The odontoid process articulates with the atlas; it occupies the anterior part of the large foramen of the atlas. This is the pivot around which the atlas and the skull rotate, allowing the shaking movements of the head.

The other cervical vertebrae (third to seventh) are typical. The third to the sixth have cleft spinous processes. A strong band runs along their spinous processes. This is called the *nuchal ligament*; it helps to support the weight of the head. The seventh cervical vertebra is known as the *vertebra prominens* as it has a prominent spinous process that may be palpated at the base of the neck.

The thoracic vertebrae

There are 12 thoracic vertebrae. These are typical; but in addition to the features described, they also have facets on their bodies and transverse processes that provide points for articulation with the ribs.

The lumbar vertebrae

The five lumbar vertebrae have the largest bodies and the smallest foramina. Their spinous processes are thicker and less pointed, but they are still easily identified in the lower part of the back.

The sacrum

Five sacral vertebrae are fused together, forming a triangular-shaped bone called the sacrum (Fig. 2.10). The anterior surface is concave; the superior part articulates with the fifth lumbar vertebra. Each side articulates with

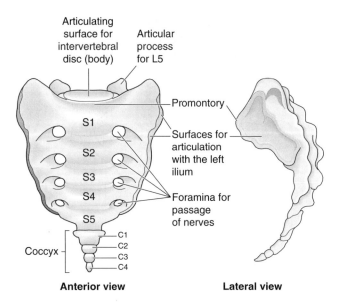

Articulating
surface for
intervertebral
disc (body)

Articular
process
for L5

S1
S2
S3
S4
S5

Promontory

Surfaces for
articulation
with the left
ilium

Foramina for
passage
of nerves

Coccyx
C1
C2
C3
C4

Anterior view   **Lateral view**

Fig. 2.10 The sacrum and the coccyx (from Waugh A, Grant A. Ross and Wilson Anatomy and physiology in health and illness. 9th edn. Edinburgh: Churchill Livingstone; 2001).

the ilium, and the lower part articulates with the coccyx. The sacrum is wedged between the innominate bones at the back of the pelvis. On each side, foramina allow the passage of nerves.

The coccyx

The last four vertebrae are fused to form a single triangular structure called the coccyx (Fig. 2.10). The coccyx has no known function in humans, but in many vertebrates it is the tail.

The functions of the vertebral column
Protection

The delicate spinal cord extends the length of the vertebral canal, from the first cervical vertebra to the lumbar region (Fig. 2.11), yet the spine can be bent and twisted causing no damage.

A series of ligaments (Fig. 2.12) holds the vertebrae together and prevents them from slipping – allowing a range of safe movement, and no more (Box 2.5). The *anterior longitudinal ligament* extends the length of the column, in front of the vertebral bodies. The *posterior longitudinal ligament* also extends the length of the column, but lies close to the bodies of the vertebrae inside the vertebral canal itself. The laminae of adjacent vertebrae are joined by the *ligamenta flava*; the *ligamentum nuchae* in the cervical region, and the *supraspinous ligament* in the thoracic and lumbar regions, join the spinous processes.

Support

The vertebral column acts as a support for the body. This is possible because of the shape of the bones, and the presence of ligaments and

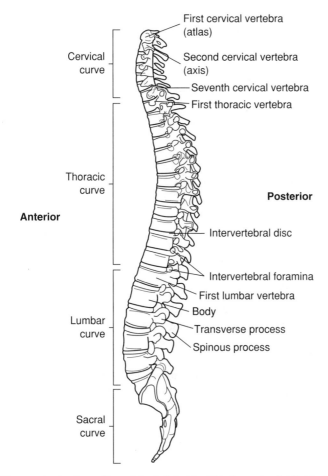

Fig. 2.11 The vertebral column (from Fritz S, Paholsky KM, Grosenbach MJ. Mosby's basic science for soft tissue and movement therapies. St Louis: Mosby; 1998).

muscles. There are groups of muscles attached to the spine for the whole of its length. These produce the movements that allow the spine to be fixed in whatever position is desired so that it may act as a rigid support.

■ BOX 2.5 Damage to the spinal cord

In injury to the back or neck these ligaments may be torn, allowing the vertebrae to move away from each other, disrupting the continuous canal and damaging the cord. The spinal cord carries the nerves from the brain to all parts of the body, so an injury to it may result in *tetraplegia* or *paraplegia*. In these conditions, there is paralysis of all the muscles below the level of the injury to the spinal cord. Thus, in the case of back or neck injury, particular care must be taken when moving the casualty – avoiding any movement of the spine.

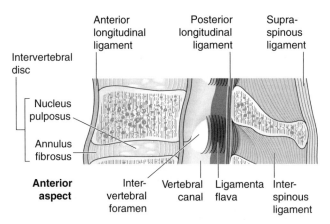

Fig. 2.12 Section of the vertebral column (from Waugh A, Grant A. Ross and Wilson Anatomy and physiology in health and illness. 9th edn. Edinburgh: Churchill Livingstone; 2001).

Axis of the trunk

The vertebral column forms the axis of the trunk, to which the ribs, shoulder girdle/upper limbs, and pelvic girdle/lower limbs are attached.

Movement

The spine is mobile, permitting a wide range of forward, backward, side to side and twisting movements. These movements are possible because there are small, freely moveable *facet joints* between the laminae of all vertebrae. Discs of specialized tissue lie between the vertebral bodies, acting as cushions or shock absorbers. These are called *intervertebral discs*.

THE SKULL

The skull is described in two parts – the cranium and the face (Figs 2.13 and 2.14).

The cranium

Eight flat and irregular bones form the cranial cavity – a protective enclosure for the brain.

1. The *frontal bone* forms the forehead and the roof of the orbits (the cone-shaped cavities which contain the eyes).
2. The two *parietal bones* form the top or vault of the cranium.
3. The two *temporal bones* contain the internal parts of the ears. On the outer surface the opening for the ear is found, and the prominent *mastoid process* is located behind this. The mastoid process is a point of attachment for some of the muscles that move the head. There are tiny air spaces in this thick portion of the bone. The *mandibular fossa* is the part of each temporal bone that articulates with the jaw, at the *temporomandibular* joint.
4. The *occipital bone* forms the posterior part of the base of the skull. It contains a large opening – the *foramen magnum* – which allows passage

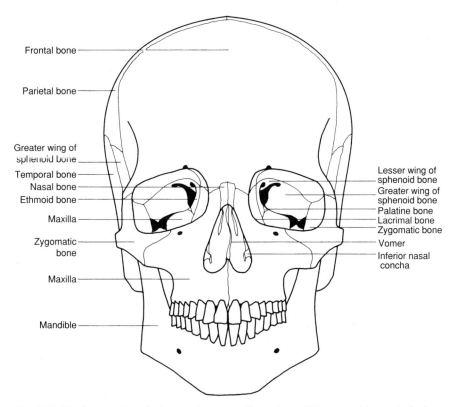

Fig. 2.13 The bones of the skull – anterior aspect (from Gunn C. Bones and joints. 3rd edn. Edinburgh: Churchill Livingstone; 1996).

of the spinal cord from the brain to the vertebral canal. On either side of the foramen magnum there are surfaces (*condylar fossa*) for articulation with the atlas.

5. The *sphenoid bone* is an irregular bone shaped like a bat. It forms part of the floor of the skull, and lies between the frontal, temporal and occipital bones. It consists of a body, two wing-like structures and two processes, the *pterygoid processes*. There are two openings, called the *optic foramina*, through which the optic nerves pass from the eyes to the brain.

6. The *ethmoid* bone is an irregular, box-shaped bone, which forms the bony framework of the nose. The superior surface, the *cribriform plate*, is perforated to allow passage of the olfactory nerve – the nerve of smell.

The face

The skeleton of the face consists of 13 irregular bones arranged in such a way that they form the orbits, part of the nose and the walls of the mouth or oral cavity.

1. The two *zygomatic bones* are the cheekbones, and they also from part of the orbits.
2. The *maxilla* is the upper jaw – the two maxillae articulate with the upper teeth and form part of the roof of the mouth.

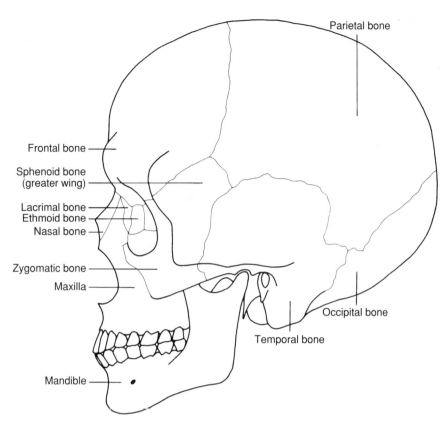

Fig. 2.14 The bones of the skull – lateral aspect (from Gunn C. Bones and joints. 3rd edn. Edinburgh: Churchill Livingstone; 1996).

3. The *mandible* is the lower jaw. It articulates with the lower teeth, and forms the freely moveable temporomandibular joints with the temporal bones.
4. The *nasal bones* are flat bones forming the bridge of the nose.
5. The *lacrimal bones* are very small irregular bones that lie on the medial walls (inner corners) of the orbits. They form passages for the tear ducts.
6. The *inferior nasal conchae* are irregular bones that form the lateral walls of the nasal cavity. These bones have a scroll-like appearance, and their name, *concha*, is derived from the Latin word for shell. The inferior nasal conchae are sometimes called *turbinates*, as their shape causes agitation, or turbulence, of the air that is breathed in through the nose.
7. The *vomer* is a flat bone that forms the posterior and inferior part of the bony nasal septum.
8. The *palatine bones* form the roof of the mouth, or palate.

The joints of the skull

The joints of the skull, with the exception of the temporomandibular joints, are immoveable joints called *sutures*. The edges of the bones are finely serrated, and they fit together like the pieces of an intricate jigsaw puzzle (Fig. 2.15).

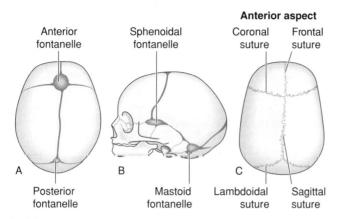

Fig. 2.15 The fontanelles and sutures of the skull. (A) Fontanelles viewed from above; (B) fontanelles viewed from the side; (C) main sutures viewed from above when ossification is complete. (From Waugh A, Grant A. Ross and Wilson Anatomy and physiology in health and illness. 9th edn. Edinburgh: Churchill Livingstone; 2001.)

In an infant, there is a soft area where the frontal and parietal bones meet. This suture does not ossify until the child is about 18 months old. This is called the *anterior fontanelle* (Fig. 2.15). It is the easiest site to take the pulse of an infant, as the pulsation of the blood vessels can be felt through the soft membrane. There is a similar fontanelle at the back of the skull, but this ossifies in the first few weeks of life. These soft areas allow the skull to be moulded during birth.

The sinuses of the skull

The *paranasal sinuses* of the skull are spaces containing air in the frontal, ethmoid and sphenoid bones, and also in the maxillae. These sinuses communicate with the nose; they lighten the skull and help with voice production and resonance.

■ BOX 2.6 Sinusitis

Spread of infection from the nose or throat to the paranasal sinuses results in a condition known as sinusitis.

THE THORAX OR THORACIC CAGE

The thorax is the superior cavity of the trunk. The 12 thoracic vertebrae described earlier form the posterior part of the thoracic cage; the ribs and costal cartilage form the lateral and anterior walls, and the sternum forms the anterior part. The thoracic cage protects the heart and the lungs, and the organs of the upper abdominal cavity.

The sternum

The *sternum* is the breastbone (Fig. 2.16). It is comprised mainly of cancellous bone tissue, thus it is very light. It is easily palpated, as it lies just

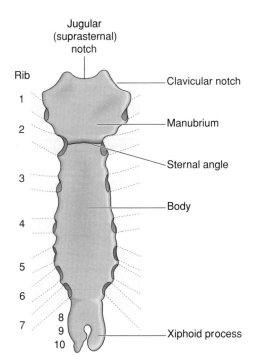

Fig. 2.16 The sternum and its attachments (from Waugh A, Grant A. Ross and Wilson Anatomy and physiology in health and illness. 9th edn. Edinburgh: Churchill Livingstone; 2001).

■ BOX 2.7 Cardiac massage

The heart lies immediately behind the body of the sternum. External cardiac massage is a means of stimulating the heart if it has stopped beating. Rhythmically pressing on the sternum massages the heart; this is carried out until the heart starts to beat on its own. When performing cardiac massage, it is important to place the 'heel' of the hand on the lower third of the body of the sternum, and not over the xiphoid process. Direct pressure here could cause the bone to break.

---

under the skin. The sternum is a dagger-shaped flat bone, and consists of three parts:

- the *manubrium* ('handle') is the superior part; it articulates with the clavicles (collar bones) and the first pair of ribs
- the *body* ('blade') is middle portion; it articulates with the ribs
- the *xiphoid process* is the pointed inferior tip of the bone; muscles of the anterior abdominal wall and the diaphragm attach here.

The ribs

There are 12 pairs of ribs. A rib is a flat, curved bone attached posteriorly to the thoracic vertebrae by the *head* and the *tubercle* (Fig. 2.17). The shaft

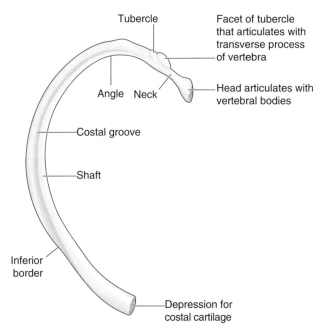

Tubercle

Facet of tubercle
that articulates with
transverse process
of vertebra

Head articulates with
vertebral bodies

Angle   Neck

Costal groove

Shaft

Inferior
border

Depression for
costal cartilage

Fig. 2.17 A typical rib viewed from below (from Waugh A, Grant A. Ross and Wilson Anatomy and physiology in health and illness. 9th edn. Edinburgh: Churchill Livingstone; 2001).

curves backwards then forwards, and it is attached to the sternum by strips of hyaline cartilage known as *costal cartilage*.

1. The first seven pairs of ribs are *true ribs*; they articulate with their corresponding thoracic vertebrae, and are joined to the sternum by *costal cartilage*.
2. The other ribs are *false ribs*. The eighth, ninth and tenth pairs have costal *cartilages*; however, they are indirectly joined to the sternum by means of the seventh costal cartilage. The last two pairs – the *floating ribs* – attach to the vertebrae posteriorly, and are embedded in muscle tissue.

The anterior and posterior attachments of the ribs are freely move-able, allowing easy upwards and outwards movements of the chest on breathing.

■ BOX 2.8 Fractures of the ribs

Costal cartilage allows for a degree of 'spring' in the thoracic cage. This helps to prevent fractures occurring as a result of a blow to the chest. However, if a blow is sufficiently violent, the ribs will fracture and this injury may then be complicated by damage to the lungs by the fractured ribs.

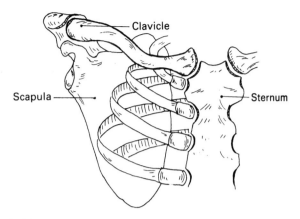

Fig. 2.18 The clavicle.

THE SHOULDER GIRDLE

The shoulder girdle consists of two *clavicles* (collar bones) and two *scapulae* (shoulder blades). These bones form an incomplete girdle around the upper part of the thorax. The function of the shoulder girdle is to give the upper limb a greater range of movement. Many movements are possible at the shoulder girdle – the clavicles control the movement at the scapulae.

The clavicle

The clavicle (Fig. 2.18) is a long bone, with an S-shaped shaft; it runs horizontally from the base of the neck to the shoulder. It is easily palpable along its entire length, from its attachment to the manubrium to the *acromial* end, at the point on the shoulder where it attaches to the scapula.

   The main function of the clavicle is to act as a strut, holding the shoulders back. Although the clavicle is a long bone, it does not have a medullary cavity. The clavicle is the first bone of the body that ossifies; it is ossified from a membrane. However, ossification is not complete until age 25.

■ BOX 2.9 **Fractures of the clavicle**

The clavicle may be fractured by a fall onto an outstretched hand; the shoulder falls forwards and downwards. The usual treatment is the application of a figure-of-eight bandage or harness – the aim being to brace the shoulder back into position until the bone heals.

The scapula

The scapula is a flat, triangular-shaped bone (Fig. 2.19). The word means a *digging tool*. The body of the scapula is formed like a large, flat blade; and the spine of the scapula projects to the back. The scapula lies between the levels of the second and seventh ribs. The body of the scapula is separated from the ribs by soft tissue and muscle; it moves on the back of the thorax,

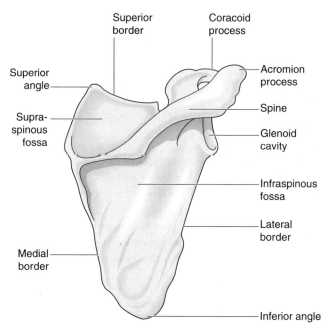

Fig. 2.19 The right scapula, posterior aspect (from Waugh A, Grant A. Ross and Wilson Anatomy and physiology in health and illness. 9th edn. Edinburgh: Churchill Livingstone; 2001).

giving the 'shrugging' movements of the shoulders. The scapula is a point of attachment for many muscles.

1. The scapular body is triangular in shape therefore has three angles (notably the *inferior* and *superior angles*) and three sides or borders (notably the *superior, medial* and *lateral borders*).
2. At the lateral end of the superior border, muscles attach to the *coracoid process.*
3. The lateral border forms one of the boundaries of the space under the arm known as the *axilla.*
4. At the superior part of the lateral border, there is a shallow, saucer-shaped surface known as the *glenoid cavity.* This is the surface that articulates with the head of the humerus, forming the shoulder joint.
5. The spine of the scapula lies just under the skin. It may be felt along its entire length, from near the midline to the lateral end where it broadens to form the *acromion process* at the junction with the clavicle.

THE UPPER LIMBS

Each upper limb consists of:

- a *humerus* in the upper arm
- a *radius* and *ulna* in the forearm
- eight *carpal bones* in the wrist
- five *metacarpals* and 14 *phalanges* of the hand and fingers.

The humerus

The humerus is a long bone; it is the longest and strongest bone of the upper limb (Fig. 2.20).

1. The upper extremity has a rounded *head* that articulates with the glenoid cavity of the scapula.
2. Lateral to the head is the *greater tubercle (tuberosity)*, a rough process for the attachment of muscles.
3. Below the upper extremity the bone narrows to form the shaft. This narrow part is called the *surgical neck*.
4. The *bicipital groove*, or *intertubercular sulcus*, lies between the greater and lesser tubercles. This is an attachment point for muscles that move the shoulder.
5. The lower end of the extremity is broader and flatter than the upper extremity. It has two articular surfaces involved in the elbow joint. The pulley-shaped *trochlea* articulates with the ulna; the rounded *capitulum* articulates with the radius.

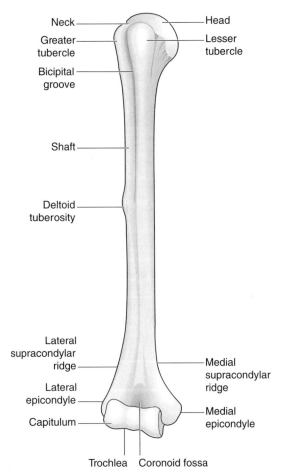

Fig. 2.20 The right humerus, anterior aspect (from Waugh A, Grant A. Ross and Wilson Anatomy and physiology in health and illness. 9th edn. Edinburgh: Churchill Livingstone; 2001).

■ BOX 2.10 Injuries to the humerus

1. The surgical neck is a site that is often fractured in shoulder injuries. This is common in elderly people.
2. The radial nerve, which supplies the muscles of the forearm, wrist and hand, winds around the back of the shaft of the humerus. Careless handling of an unconscious patient, or incorrect use of crutches, may damage this nerve and result in a 'dropped wrist'.

6. Two rounded projections, *epicondyles*, are palpable at the lower end of the humerus. The ulnar nerve winds round the back of the *medial epicondyle* – if it is compressed against the bone a tingling sensation is produced, hence the term 'funny bone'.

The radius

The radius is the lateral bone of the forearm. It is joined to the ulna by an *interosseous membrane* at its medial border. In the anatomical position, it is the bone in line with the thumb. It is a long bone.

1. The proximal extremity has a disc-shaped *head* that articulates not only with the humerus at the elbow joint but also with the ulna, allowing rotating movements of the forearm (Fig. 2.21).
2. The *radial tuberosity* may be felt on the medial side.
3. The distal end is larger and flatter in form. It articulates with two of the carpal bones (the lunate and scaphoid) at the wrist joint, and also with the distal extremity of the ulna.
4. The *styloid process* (pen-shaped) is located on the distal, lateral side of the radius.

The ulna

The ulna is the medial bone of the forearm. It is a long bone with a claw-shaped proximal extremity that articulates with the humerus and the radius (Fig. 2.21).

1. The *olecranon* or *olecranon process* is the prominence felt at the elbow.
2. The distal end of the ulna consists of a small rounded *head* that articulates with the carpus and the radius. The *ulnar styloid process* projects from this head on the posterior end. The head of the ulna can be seen at the back of the wrist in line with the little finger.

The carpal bones

The *carpus* (wrist) is composed of eight small, short bones arranged roughly in two rows of four (Fig. 2.22). There is free gliding movement between

■ BOX 2.11 Feeling a pulse

The radial artery passes over the anterior surface of the radius, just below the thumb. This is the most convenient site at which to feel the pulse.

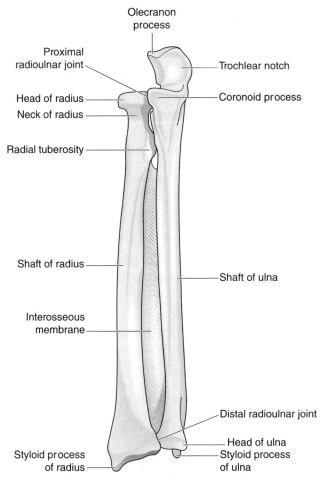

Fig. 2.21 The right radius and ulna, anterior aspect (from Waugh A, Grant A. Ross and Wilson Anatomy and physiology in health and illness. 9th edn. Edinburgh: Churchill Livingstone; 2001).

the bones. This arrangement allows flexibility at the wrist, but it is also a strong structure that can take the weight of the body.

1. The *proximal* row of bones articulates with the radius and ulna. The bones are named (from the radial side to the ulnar side) the *scaphoid, lunate, triquetral* and *pisiform*.
2. The *distal* row of bones articulates with the metacarpals. The bones are named (from the radial side to the ulnar side) the *trapezium, trapezoid, capitate* and *hamate*.

The metacarpals

The *metacarpals* are five miniature long bones located in the palm region of each hand (Fig. 2.22). They are numbered for identification, from 1 to 5, from lateral to medial. The first metacarpal forms the base of the thumb. The rounded heads form the knuckles, which articulate with the phalanges that form the fingers.

■ **BOX 2.12 Carpal tunnel syndrome**

Tendons of muscles of the forearm cross the carpus. Strong bands of fibrous tissue known as the *retinacula* hold them close to the bones. Some of the carpals and the *flexor retinaculum* (anterior surface of the wrist) form the *carpal tunnel*. The *median nerve* passes through this structure; if this is compressed due to trauma, swelling or repetitive flexion of the wrist, *carpal tunnel syndrome* may develop.

The phalanges

The *phalanges* are also miniature long bones. There are 14 in total in each hand – three in each finger and two in the thumb (Fig. 2.22). Each finger has a *proximal, middle* and *distal phalanx*. The thumb is known as the *pollux*, and does not have a middle phalanx.

THE PELVIC GIRDLE

The pelvic girdle is comprised of two fused bones, the *innominate* bone and the sacrum. This unit forms the pelvic cavity, which contains the organs of reproduction. The formation of the female pelvis differs from that of the

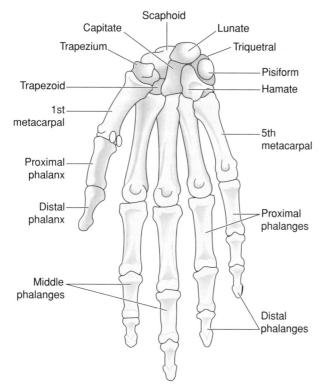

Fig. 2.22 The bones of the wrist, hand and fingers, anterior aspect (from Waugh A, Grant A. Ross and Wilson Anatomy and physiology in health and illness. 9th edn. Edinburgh: Churchill Livingstone; 2001).

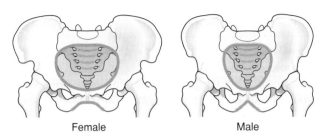

Female   Male

Fig. 2.23 The female and male pelves (from Waugh A, Grant A. Ross and Wilson Anatomy and physiology in health and illness. 9th edn. Edinburgh: Churchill Livingstone; 2001).

male. The male pelvis is smaller, narrower and more funnel-shaped than the female pelvis, which is larger, wider and more cylindrical in shape (Fig. 2.23).

The lower limbs carry the weight of the body; therefore the pelvic girdle must provide a strong and stable support.

The innominate bone

Three bones fuse together during childhood to form the *innominate* bone (Fig. 2.24). The upper part is flat, the remainder irregular in form. The bones are the *ilium*, the *ischium* and the *pubis*.

1. The *ilium* is the flat upper part of the innominate bone. It is a point of attachment for the powerful hip muscles. At the superior part of the ilium, there is a thick curved crest (the *iliac crest*) that can be felt just below the waist. The anterior and posterior parts of the crest end in spines, the *anterior superior iliac spine* and the *posterior superior iliac spine*. Below the posterior superior iliac spine is the *great sciatic notch*, where the sciatic nerve emerges from the pelvis and enters the region of the buttock.
2. The *ischium* is the inferior and posterior portion. On each side, there is a large prominence, the *ischial tuberosity*, which takes the weight of the body when seated. These tuberosities are protected by small, fluid-filled sacs known as *bursae*, which act as cushions.
3. The pubis forms the inferior and anterior part. The two pubic bones join anteriorly at the *symphysis pubis*, which is just anterior to the bladder.

All three parts of the innominate bone unite at the cup-shaped *acetabulum*. This is the rounded cavity that receives the head of the femur to form the hip joint. Below the acetabulum there is a large opening called the *obturator foramen*. This provides a passage for the obturator nerve (which supplies medial muscles and skin) of the lower limb, and also reduces the weight of the pelvic girdle.

■ **BOX 2.13 Fractures of the pelvis**

Severe blows, such as those in road traffic accidents, can fracture the pelvis. Such fractures often result in damage to the bladder, urethra and major blood vessels.

A

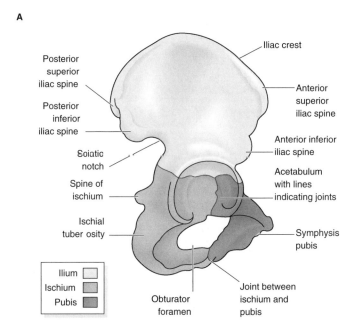

Iliac crest

Posterior superior iliac spine

Posterior inferior iliac spine

Sciatic notch

Spine of ischium

Ischial tuber osity

Anterior superior iliac spine

Anterior inferior iliac spine

Acetabulum with lines indicating joints

Symphysis pubis

Ilium

Ischium

Pubis

Obturator foramen

Joint between ischium and pubis

B

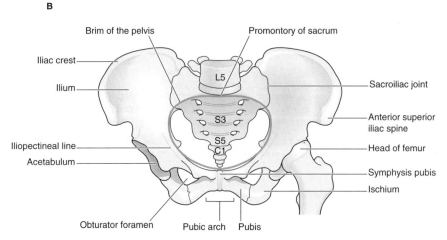

Brim of the pelvis

Promontory of sacrum

Iliac crest

Ilium

Iliopectineal line

Acetabulum

L5

S3

S5

C1

Sacroiliac joint

Anterior superior iliac spine

Head of femur

Symphysis pubis

Ischium

Obturator foramen

Pubic arch

Pubis

Fig. 2.24 (A) The right innominate bone, lateral aspect. (B) The bones of the pelvis. (From Waugh A, Grant A. Ross and Wilson Anatomy and physiology in health and illness. 9th edn. Edinburgh: Churchill Livingstone; 2001).

THE LOWER LIMBS

Each lower limb consists of

- a *femur* – the thigh bone
- a *tibia* and a *fibula* in the lower leg
- *tarsal* bones at the ankle and foot
- *metacarpals* and *phalanges* of the foot and toes.

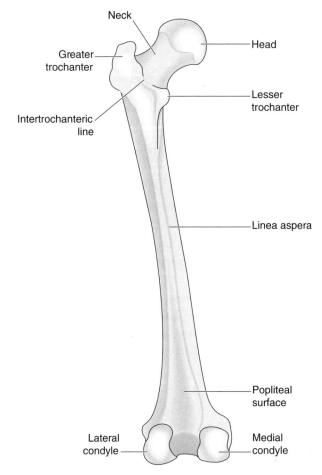

Fig. 2.25 The left femur, posterior aspect (from Waugh A, Grant A. Ross and Wilson Anatomy and physiology in health and illness. 9th edn. Edinburgh: Churchill Livingstone; 2001).

The femur

The femur is the longest, strongest and heaviest bone in the body (Fig. 2.25).

1. Proximally, a rounded head fits in to the acetabulum, forming the 'ball and socket' hip joint. The head is connected to the shaft by a narrow, angled neck.
2. Lateral to the neck lies the important bony landmark, the *greater trochanter*, which along with the inferior, medially placed, *lesser trochanter* gives attachment to many muscles.
3. The shaft of the femur is long and curved slightly forwards. It ends in two rounded condyles, the *medial* and *lateral condyles*, that articulate with the tibia, forming the knee joint.
4. Superior to these condyles, *medial* and *lateral epicondyles* give attachment to ligaments.

■ **BOX 2.14 The neck of the femur**

A fracture to the neck of the femur, caused by falling, is a fairly common injury in elderly females.

'Bow legs' and 'knock knees' are a consequence of abnormal angulations of the neck of the femur.

5. The smooth *patellar articular surface* is located on the anterior surface between the condyles.
6. On the posterior aspect the triangular *popliteal surface* borders the *popliteal space* behind the knee, where blood vessels and nerves pass to the lower leg.

The patella

The *patella*, or kneecap (Fig. 2.26), is a sesamoid bone, a type of short bone that develops in the tendon of a muscle. The triangular patella is located in the tendons of the *quadriceps femoris*, which crosses the knee joint. It takes the weight in the kneeling position. Like the ischial tuberosity, it is protected by a small bursa.

■ **BOX 2.15**

The patella is absent in babies, appearing between the ages of 3 and 6 years. Ossification is complete at puberty.

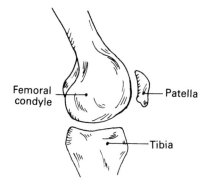

Femoral condyle — Patella — Tibia

Relationship between patella and femur

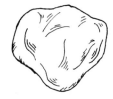

The patella

Fig. 2.26 The patella and its relationship to the femur.

The tibia

The tibia, or shinbone (Fig. 2.27), is the medial bone of the lower leg. It is a long bone. It is thicker than the fibula, and is the weight-bearing bone.

1. The expanded proximal extremity consists of two prominent *condyles*. These articulate with the femoral condyles at the knee joint.
2. The tibia has a facet on the inferior surface of the lateral condyle that articulates with the head of the fibula.
3. The *tibial tuberosity*, palpable on the anterior surface just below the condyles, gives attachment to the patellar ligament.
4. The *shaft* of the tibia is triangular in section, with a subcutaneous *anterior border* – the *tibial crest*, or shin.
5. At the distal end, the prominent medial projection is the *medial malleolus* that helps form the ankle joint.
6. The inferior posterior surface of the tibia articulates with the *talus* bone of the foot.

The fibula

The fibula (Fig. 2.27) is the lateral bone of the lower leg. It is thinner than the tibia, it does not bear weight as it does not articulate directly with the knee joint, and it may be distorted by the pull of muscles. It is a

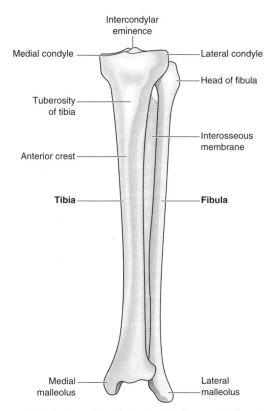

Fig. 2.27 The tibia and fibula (from Waugh A, Grant A. Ross and Wilson Anatomy and physiology in health and illness. 9th edn. Edinburgh: Churchill Livingstone; 2001).

■ **BOX 2.16 The head of the fibula**

The head of the fibula may be felt on the outside of the knee, slightly towards the back. The important *common peroneal nerve* winds around this prominence. This nerve is easily damaged by pressure. As it supplies the muscles that produce dorsiflexion and eversion at the foot and ankle, injury to it will cause 'drop foot'. Thus great care must be taken to avoid inflicting pressure over this area.

point of attachment for many muscles and fascia, and acts as a lateral splint for the ankle. The fibula can withstand more tensile strain than any other bone.

1. The proximal extremity is the knob-like head, which articulates with the inferior surface of the lateral tibial condyle.
2. The shaft of the fibula is joined along its length to the tibia by an *interosseous membrane*.
3. The distal extremity is the *lateral malleolus*. This is the easily palpated, outer bone of the ankle. The distal end articulates with the talus.

The tarsus

The structure of the foot is similar to that of the hand; however, as it is weight bearing, the foot needs to be stronger but not as mobile. Its structure reflects its functions – there are 26 bones, 31 joints and more than 20 muscles in the foot.

Seven tarsal bones comprise the posterior part of the foot (Fig. 2.28).

1. The *talus* forms the ankle joint with the tibia and fibula. It is the major weight-bearing bone of the foot. It articulates inferiorly with the calcaneus.
2. The *calcaneus* is the largest bone of the foot. It projects backwards and forms the heel.

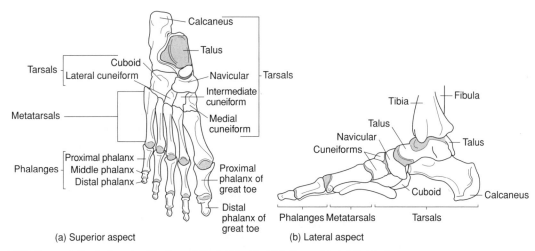

Fig. 2.28 Bones of the foot and ankle (from Fritz S, Paholsky KM, Grosenbach MJ. Mosby's basic science for soft tissue and movement therapies. St Louis: Mosby; 1998).

3. The *navicular* bone is disc-shaped, with three facets that articulate with the cuneiform bones.
4. The three *cuneiforms* are wedge-shaped, and named the *medial, intermediate* and *lateral cuneiform* bones.
5. The *cuboid* is a flattened, six-sided bone that articulates with the talus. The lateral and inferior surface has a deep groove for the *peroneus longus* tendon.

The metatarsals

The five metatarsal bones form the 'instep' of the foot. They are miniature long bones that are located distal to the tarsus (Fig. 2.28). They are numbered medially to laterally from one to five. The heads of the metatarsals form the 'ball' of the foot.

1. The first metatarsal is shorter and thicker than the others and has two facets on the plantar aspect of its head for sesamoid bones.
2. The second metatarsal is the longest.
3. The fifth metatarsal has a tuberosity that projects directly from the base.

The phalanges

The phalanges are miniature long bones that lie distal to the metatarsals. Fourteen phalanges form the toes on each foot. The arrangement is similar to that found in the fingers:

- the big toe, or hallux, has two phalanges
- the other toes have each a proximal, middle and distal phalanx.

A thorough knowledge of the bony structure of the foot, coupled with skills of palpation, is essential for the practice of reflexology.

■ BOX 2.17 The arches of the foot

The bones of the foot are arranged in such a way that they form three arches, two lengthwise and one across the foot. These arches give the foot its 'spring'. If they fall (e.g. due to muscular weakness and the consequent stretching of ligaments), the gait will be ungainly and the feet will be painful.

The *plantar aponeurosis* is a band of connective tissue that extends along the plantar surface of the foot, from the inferior aspect of the calcaneus to the toes. It adds stability to the arches.

1. The *medial longitudinal arch* is the highest of the arches. It is formed by the calcaneus, navicular, three cuneiforms and the first three metatarsals. Only the calcaneus and the distal parts of the metatarsals should be in contact with the ground when standing. The *plantar calcaneonavicular* ligament, or '*spring ligament*' is important in supporting the medial longitudinal arch.
2. The *lateral longitudinal arch* is less pronounced. It is formed by the calcaneus, cuboid, and fourth and fifth metatarsals.
3. The metatarsal heads form the *transverse arch*.

THE SKELETAL SYSTEM QUESTIONS

Diagrams—Questions 36–86

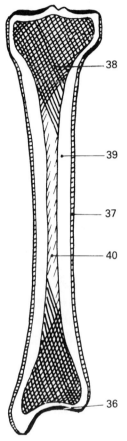

36–40. Diagram of a long bone

A. Red bone marrow
B. Compact bone tissue
C. Hyaline cartilage
D. Medullary canal
E. Periosteum

36
37
38
39
40

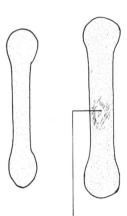 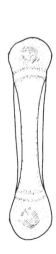 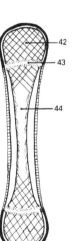 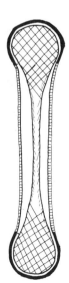

41–44. Diagram of a growing bone

A. Epiphysis
B. Diaphysis
C. Epiphyseal cartilage
D. Primary centre of ossification

41
42
43
44

45–50. A vertebra

A. Body
B. Lamina
C. Pedicle
D. Neural arch
E. Spinous process
F. Vertebral foramen

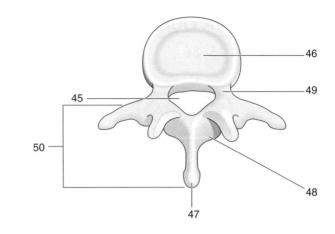

45 _____
46 _____
47 _____
48 _____
49 _____
50 _____

51–57. The skull

A. Temporal bone
B. Frontal bone
C. Lacrimal bone
D. Maxilla
E. Mandible
F. Nasal bones
G. Zygomatic bone

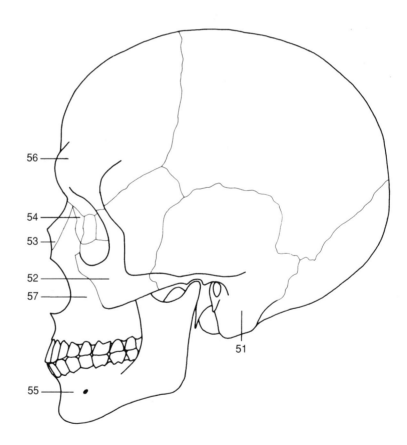

51 _____
52 _____
53 _____
54 _____
55 _____
56 _____
57 _____

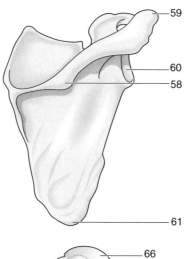

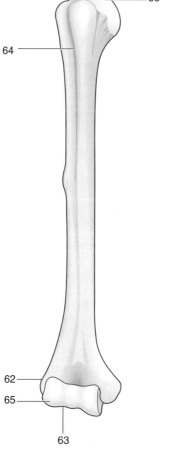

58–61. **The scapula**

A. Acromion process
B. Inferior angle
C. Glenoid cavity
D. Spine

58
59
60
61

62–66. **The humerus**

A. Capitulum
B. Head
C. Lateral
   epicondyle
D. Bicipital groove
E. Trochlea

62
63
64
65
66

67–70. The radius and ulna

A. Distal radioulnar joint
B. Head of radius
C. Head of ulna
D. Olecranon process

67
68
69
70

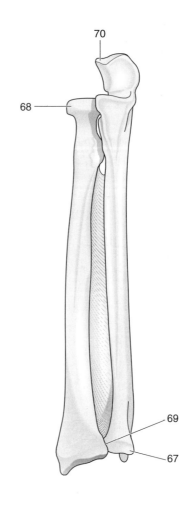

71–75. The innominate bone

A. Acetabulum
B. Ischial tuberosity
C. Iliac crest
D. Sciatic notch
E. Symphysis pubis

71
72
73
74
75

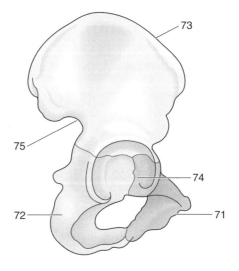

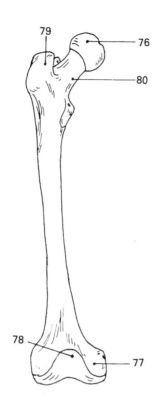

76–80. The femur

A. Head
B. Neck
C. Greater
   trochanter
D. Medial condyle
E. Patellar surface

76
77
78
79
80

81–86. The tibia, fibula and foot

A. Calcaneus
B. Head of fibula
C. Medial condyle of tibia
D. Medial malleolus
E. Talus
F. Anterior crest

| 81 |
| 82 |
| 83 |
| 84 |
| 85 |
| 86 |

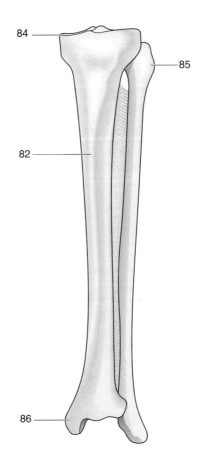

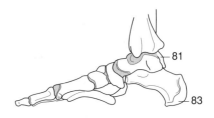

Questions 87–95 are of the multiple choice type

87. Which one of the following statements describes the term proximal?   87
A. Away from the midline
B. Near the midline
C. Nearest to the body
D. Palm down.

88. Which one of the following describes a foramen in a bone? It is: 88
A. a groove
B. a hole
C. a notch
D. a smooth surface.

89. Living bone tissue consists of one of the following: 89
A. 5% water
B. 25% water
C. 90% solids
D. 50% solids.

90. The number of lumbar vertebrae is: 90
A. 12
B. 7
C. 5
D. 4

91. Which one of the following statements describes the parietal bones? They: 91
A. contain the foramen magnum
B. form the orbits
C. are part of the face
D. are part of the cranium.

92. The mastoid process is a part of one of the following bones. Which one?   92
A. Frontal
B. Occipital
C. Sphenoid
D. Temporal.

93. The nerve of smell passes through one of the following bones. Which one?   93
A. Ethmoid
B. Frontal
C. Nasal
D. Sphenoid.

94. The ribs are classified as: 94
A. Long bones
B. Flat bones
C. Short bones
D. Irregular bones.

95. The bones of the thumb are classified as:

A. Long bones

B. Flat bones

C. Short bones

D. Irregular bones.

Questions 96–111 are of the true/false type   T | F

96–99. The growth of bone tissue is influenced by:
    96. the amount of calcium in the diet
    97. the amount of iron in the diet
    98. the amount of vitamin B in the diet
    99. the endocrine glands.

100–103. The term supine means:
    100. lying face down
    101. lying face up
    102. palm down
    103. palm up.

104–107. The cervical curve is:
    104. a primary curve
    105. a secondary curve
    106. concave backwards
    107. concave forwards.

108–111. The xiphoid process is:
    108. a part of one of the bones of the face
    109. the attachment of the eleventh rib
    110. part of the sternum
    111. anterior to the heart.

Questions 112–120 are of the matching items type

112–114. From the list on the left select the anatomical part which forms the structure on the right.

A. Acromion process	112. Funny bone	112
B. Greater trochanter	113. Knuckles	113
C. Heads of the metacarpals	114. Point of elbow.	114
D. Medial epicondyle		
E. Olecranon process		

115–117. From the list on the left select the anatomical part which is formed by the structure on the right.

A. Calcaneus	115. Heel	115
B. Patella	116. Knee cap	116
C. Talus	117. Shin.	117
D. Tibial crest		
E. Tibial condyle		

118–120. From the list on the left select the site where damage might result in the development of the condition on the right.

A. Lateral aspect of the knee	118. Dropped wrist	118
B. Medial malleolus	119. Dropped foot	119
C. Pelvis	120. Paraplegia.	120
D. Shaft of humerus		
E. Vertebral column		

The joints

3

■ KEY POINTS

- Joint structure
- Connective tissue components: collagen, elastin, bursae, cartilage
- Joint categories

- Terminology: general and specific joint movements
- Range of motion
- Major joints of the body
- Common joint disorders.

INTRODUCTION

Arthrology is the study of the joints – the articulations between the bones. The soft-tissue and movement therapies, including therapeutic and remedial massage, sports therapy, but also osteopathy and chiropractic medicine, interact most directly with the muscles, connective tissue, bones and joints. Therefore, practitioners of these therapeutic disciplines require a thorough understanding of both the anatomy and physiology of the joints.

A joint is a junction between two or more bones. Joints may be simple or complex, and their functions are determined by their structural design. Joints provide stability, static support and mobility.

CONNECTIVE TISSUE COMPONENTS

All joints have connective tissue components. These can be joint capsules, ligaments, tendons, or bursae and cartilage in some cases.

Dense fibrous tissue

The dense fibrous tissue associated with joints is composed of collagen and elastin. Collagen is predominant in white fibrous tissue, while elastin predominates in yellow fibrous tissue. Collagen has tensile strength, and is therefore important for stability, required in ligaments joining *bone to bone*. Elastin has elastic properties, allowing for stretch and recoil – crucial for mobility required in tendons, joining *muscle to bone*. The ratio of collagen to elastin in the dense fibrous tissue will determine the degrees of tensile strength and elasticity of the various tissues that comprise joint capsules, ligaments and tendons.

Ligaments and tendons

Ligaments and tendons are surrounded by loose areolar connective tissue. This forms a protective sheath.

Bursae

Bursae are sac-like structures. Their main component is *synovial* membrane, which secretes synovial fluid, a thick, sticky substance resembling raw egg white. Bursae are located, for example, between tendon and bone, to reduce friction.

Cartilage

White fibrocartilage is composed principally of collagen, and is found in joints that have stability and/or limitation of movement as their primary functions; it also forms the intervertebral discs and the menisci in the knee joints.

Hyaline cartilage, composed of water and protein, has a stiff, gel-like consistency. It covers the ends of the bones that form freely moveable joints. Hyaline cartilage reduces friction, distributes stress and absorbs pressure. Synovial fluid nourishes hyaline cartilage.

CLASSIFICATION OF JOINTS

Joints may be classified into three groups, according to *structure* and *type of movement*.

> ### ■ BOX 3.1 Classification of joints
>
> | Synarthroses | Fibrous or immovable |
> |---|---|
> | | Cartilaginous or slightly moveable |
> | Diarthroses | Synovial or freely moveable |

Fibrous joints

In a fibrous joint, the opposing edges of the bones are joined together by dense fibrous tissue, which is continuous with the periosteum. This fixes the joint, so that no movement is possible.

Examples of fibrous joints are:

1. *Sutures* (Fig. 3.1), where the bones are joined by thin ligaments, e.g. the coronal suture, the sagittal suture. In adults, there is little or no movement.
2. *Syndesmoses*, where the bones are joined by an interosseous ligament or membrane, e.g. the tibiofibular articulation, between the shaft of the tibia and fibula, and the radioulnar articulation, between the radius and ulna.

Cranio-sacral technique is thought to affect these sutures, and seeks to balance the cranial/sacral rhythm.

Cartilaginous joints

The cartilaginous joints are held either by white fibrocartilage or hyaline growth cartilage. In this case the cartilage can be compressed, and this allows slight movement.

Examples in this category include:

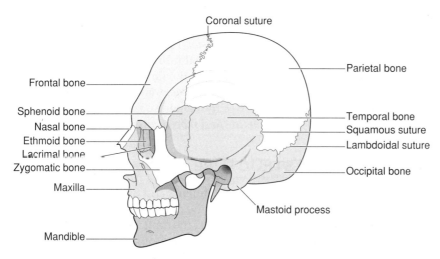

Fig. 3.1 The bones of the skull and their sutures (from Waugh A, Grant A. Ross and Wilson Anatomy and physiology in health and illness. 9th edn. Edinburgh: Churchill Livingstone; 2001).

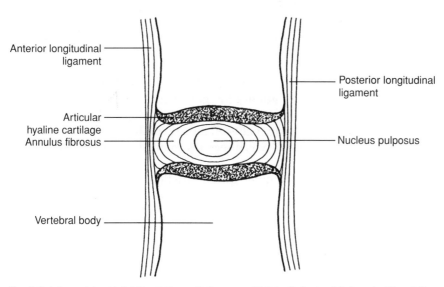

Fig. 3.2 Intervertebral joint (from Gunn C. Bones and joints. 3rd edn. Edinburgh: Churchill Livingstone; 1996).

1. *Symphysis*, e.g. the symphysis pubis, where both stability and bone union is very important. In this instance, the hyaline cartilage lines the articulating bones that are separated by thick plates of fibrocartilage. Another significant example is the joints between the vertebrae (Fig. 3.2), where shock absorption and flexibility are important.
2. *Synchondrosis*, e.g. the first sternocostal joint, where the bones are joined by hyaline growth cartilage. This ossifies in adulthood, and converts to a type of bony union known as *synostoses*. The sternocostal joint is stable, allowing only a small degree of movement.

Synovial joints

The name is derived from the Latin *syn* (like) and *ovum* (egg), which describes the sticky, viscous, clear fluid that lubricates these joints.

The main synovial joints are the joints of the limbs, and the shoulder and pelvic girdles. Synovial joints are *freely moveable*, and can be fairly complex structures allowing a wide variety of movements. Thus, synovial joints are classified according to their *structure* and *movements*.

SYNOVIAL JOINT STRUCTURE

1. In synovial joints, a joint capsule, ligaments and tendons connect the articulating bones. The joint capsule: the outer layer, known as the *stratum fibrosum*, completely surrounds the ends of the bones and is continuous with the periosteum. It has numerous sensory receptors. The inner part is the *stratum synovium*, which produces collagen, and is an entry point for nutrients and an exit point for wastes – it is highly vascular. The joint capsule also provides passive tension, which contributes to joint stability.
2. The ligaments also provide stability, keeping the articulating surfaces together by passive tension. Some ligaments may be located within the joint, e.g. the cruciate ligaments of the knee joint; however, most are extracapsular.
3. Associated muscle tendons also provide stability and, in conjunction with the ligaments, they guide joint movement.
4. Articular cartilage covers the end of the articulating bones.
5. The joint cavity is the space between the articulating bones. It is lined with synovial membrane, which secretes small amounts of synovial fluid into the cavity. This viscous fluid acts as a lubricant, allowing the surfaces to move on each other without friction.
6. Accessory structures may include fibrocartilagenous discs, plates and menisci. Along with the synovial fluid, these will prevent excessive compression of the opposing joint surfaces.

A typical synovial joint is illustrated in Figure 3.3.

MOVEMENTS AT SYNOVIAL JOINTS

Specific terms are used to describe the movements of synovial joints; these are described in Table 3.1 and illustrated in Figure 3.4.

CLASSIFICATION OF SYNOVIAL JOINTS

Synovial gliding or plane joints

These are composed of bones with flat surfaces that slide on each other, thus a gliding motion, in various planes, is permitted (Fig. 3.5). Examples of plane joints are:

- the joints between the neural arches of the vertebrae

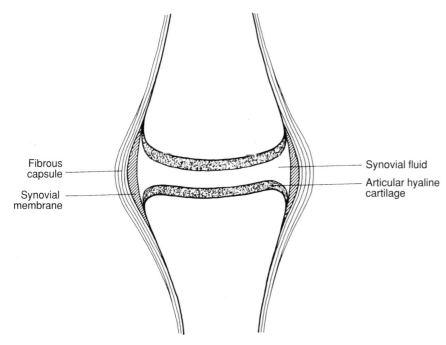

Fibrous capsule

Synovial membrane

Synovial fluid

Articular hyaline cartilage

Fig. 3.3 Typical synovial joint (from Gunn C. Bones and joints. 3rd edn. Edinburgh: Churchill Livingstone; 1996).

■ BOX 3.2 Traumatic injuries – sprains and dislocations

Sprains occur if the trauma causes damage to the fibres of ligaments. Pain, swelling and inflammation will result. Sprains can range from mild, where only a few fibres are torn, to severe, when the ligament(s) is badly damaged. Severe sprains will usually involve damage to other tissues associated with the joint, such as the joint capsule itself, tendons and accessory structures, e.g. articular cartilage, discs, menisci. If a ligament is torn, it may also result in *dislocation* or displacement (subluxation) of the joint surfaces.

Most sprains are treated by immobilization; however, pain will limit movement anyway. Prolonged immobilization can lead to contractures and weakness.

Ligamentous laxity, and reduction in the joint's stability are possible consequences of moderate and severe sprains.

■ BOX 3.3 Bursitis

Friction is generated when a tendon moves repeatedly over a bursa, and the bursa then becomes inflamed. Synovial fluid is secreted into the bursa, and it becomes swollen and tender. Bursitis at the knee joint is most common, giving rise to colloquial names to describe the location of the affected bursa, e.g. 'housemaid's knee', 'carpet layer's knee', and 'baker's cyst'.

RICE: Rest, **I**ce, **C**ompression and **E**levation
At the time of injury, it is very important that the correct first aid procedure is followed, as this will have a direct influence on the prognosis. In moderate and severe sprains, the affected part should be treated with ice, it should be compressed and elevated to limit swelling and reduce tissue fluid pressure. Medical advice should be sought immediately.

Massage is contraindicated in the initial stages of the healing process. However, in combination with rehabilitation exercises and other modalities, it can play an important part in recovery.

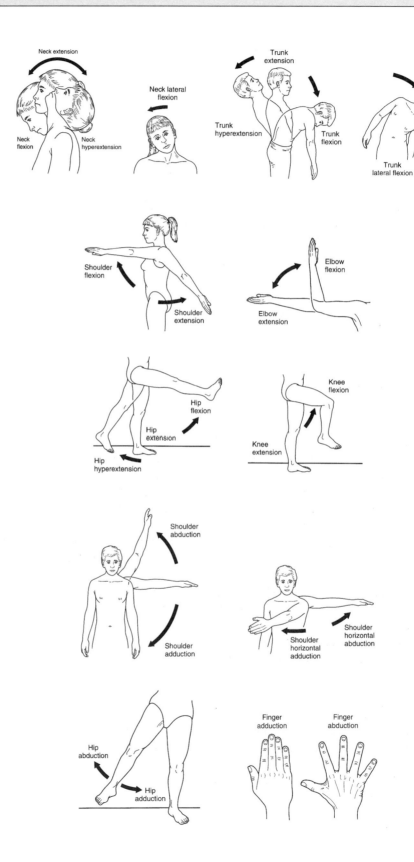

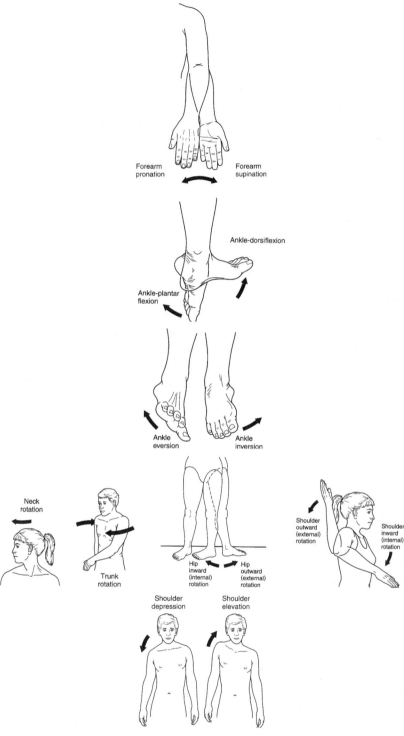

Fig. 3.4 Types of movement (from Salvo SG. Massage therapy: principles and practice. Philadelphia: WB Saunders; 1999).

■ BOX 3.4 Damage to menisci

The menisci (fibrocartilage discs) within the knee joint can be injured if the knee joint is subjected to indirect violence, usually under the conditions of bending, bearing weight and rotating. The medial meniscus is more commonly damaged, always in conjunction to damage to the medial collateral ligament and the joint capsule. This is a fairly common sports injury, and sports therapists may be involved in the rehabilitation process.

Damage to the menisci can also occur in the elderly, usually due to deep knee flexion coupled with degenerative joint changes.

Chondritis is the name given to inflammation of articular cartilage.

Massage is contraindicated in inflammatory conditions, thus it should be avoided during the 'flare ups' that often characterize rheumatoid arthritis. However, therapeutic massage and aromatherapy, for pain and stress reduction, can be very beneficial for sufferers. Carefully supervised exercise and movement therapy are also indicated.

■ BOX 3.5 Rheumatoid arthritis

Rheumatoid arthritis is an inflammatory disease affecting the synovial membrane. It is an autoimmune disorder, where the body produces antibodies that attack normal body tissues – in this case the synovial membrane. The cause is not fully understood. The synovial membrane becomes progressively inflamed, excessive quantities of synovial fluid accumulate in the joint space, and the joint becomes swollen. In time, the hyaline cartilage erodes, adhesions develop in the joint space and eventually the affected bones can become fused, resulting in complete loss of function. Any joint can be affected, but it is most common in the hands and feet.

- the sacroiliac joint
- the superior tibiofibular joint
- the acromioclavicular joint
- the costovertebral joints.

Synovial hinge joints

Hinge joints operate on one axis only (Fig. 3.5). The only possible movements are flexion and extension, in one direction. Examples of hinge joints are:

- the elbow joint
- the interphalangeal joints
- the ankle (talocrural) joint.

Often the knee is classed as a synovial hinge joint. However, as a degree of medial and lateral rotation is possible, it is in fact a condyloid joint. It is also referred to as a modified hinge joint.

The ankle joint, where dorsiflexion and plantarflexion are the only true movements possible, is also classed as a synovial hinge. However, the tibiotalar joint is a *saddle* joint, and the inferior tibiofibular joint is a fibrous *syndesmosis* joining the tibia and fibula. Thus the bones of the tarsus gliding over one another produce the other movements possible at the ankle – inversion and eversion.

Synovial pivot joints

Pivot joints allow rotation around the axis of one of the articulating bones, one of which takes the form of a ring, and the other is shaped to fit within the ring (Fig. 3.5). Examples of pivot joints are:

- the atlanto-axial joint (first and second cervical vertebrae), which permits rotating, turning or shaking movements of the head
- the proximal and distal radioulnar joints, which allow the radius to rotate over the ulna, giving the movements of pronation and supination.

Synovial condyloid joints

Condyloid joints allow movement in two planes, but one will dominate. Examples of condyloid joints are:

1. The temporomandibular joint, where opening, closing and chewing movements at the mouth are produced.
2. The wrist (radiocarpal) joint, allowing palmar flexion, extension (dorsiflexion), radial and ulnar deviation. The ulna joins the wrist indirectly via a disc, allowing pronation and supination to occur independently of any wrist movements.
3. The metacarpophalangeal and metatarsophalangeal joints allow flexion and extension, and when the fingers and toes are extended, abduction and adduction.
4. The knee joint is a complicated joint. Flexion, extension and a small degree of medial and lateral rotation are possible.

Synovial saddle joints

Saddle joints (Fig. 3.5) are less common. They are named so because their structure resembles a rider on a saddle, and because of this structure, flexion, extension, abduction, adduction and a small degree of rotation is possible. The most obvious example of a saddle joint is the carpometacarpal joint of the thumb, between the wrist and the metacarpal bone of the thumb. Here, the additional movements of rotation and circumduction are possible, and the thumb can also be opposed to the other fingers producing grasping movements.

RANGE OF MOTION AT SYNOVIAL JOINTS

Anatomic range of motion (ROM) is the range of movement that is possible at a joint; it is defined and limited by its bony structure and soft-tissue components.

However, in some joints, physiological factors will also limit the ROM. For example, sensory receptors in the joint capsule will transmit information to the nervous system, which in turn will set limits on the ROM. This is to protect and prevent injury to the joint. These limits are called the *physiologic range of motion*.

Table 3.1 General and specific joint movements

	Definition
General terms:	
Flexion	Decreases the angle between two bones, bending
Extension	Increases the angle between two bones, straightening
Abduction (can also be horizontal, diagonal)	Moving away from the midline
Adduction (can also be horizontal, diagonal)	Moving towards the midline
Circumduction	Movement in a circular direction
Rotation (medial or lateral)	Movement around a central axis
Terms specific to forearm, wrist, thumb, ankle, foot:	
Pronation	Movement of the hand/foot that turns the palm/sole in a posterior direction, i.e. so that palm faces downward or sole faces outward
Supination	Movement of the hand so that palm faces upward, or the foot so that sole faces inward
Radial flexion or deviation	Movement of the wrist in a lateral direction
Ulnar flexion or deviation	Movement of the wrist in a medial direction
Opposition of thumb	Movement of the thumb diagonally across the palmar aspect of the hand towards the fingers
Eversion	Movement of the sole of the foot away from the midline
Inversion	Movement of the sole toward the midline
Dorsiflexion	Movement at the ankle joint where the sole of the foot is moved upward, towards the anterior
Plantarflexion	Movement at the ankle joint where the sole of the foot is moved downward, towards the posterior
Terms specific to the shoulder girdle and joint:	
Elevation	Movement of the shoulder gridle in an upward direction, e.g. 'shrugging'
Depression	Movement of the shoulder girdle in an inferior direction
Protraction	Movement of the shoulder girdle in an anterior direction, scapula in abduction
Retraction	Movement of the shoulder girdle in a posterior direction, scapula adducted
Rotation downward	Movement of the scapula where its inferior angle moves medially and in a downward direction, and the acromion process moves down
Rotation upward	Movement of the scapula where its inferior angle moves laterally and upward, and the acromion process moves upward
Terms specific to the spine:	
Lateral flexion	Side bending – movement of the head or trunk laterally, away from the midline
Reduction	The spine returns to the anatomic position after lateral flexion

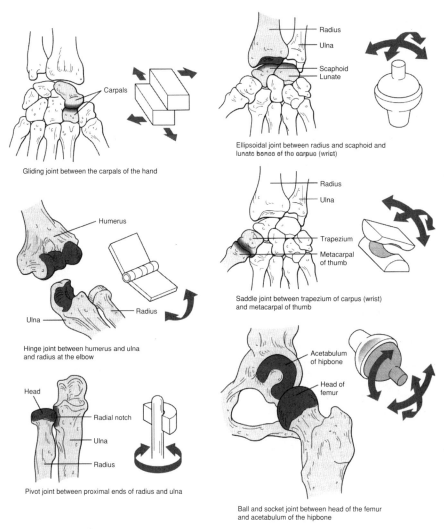

Gliding joint between the carpals of the hand

Ellipsoidal joint between radius and scaphoid and lunate bones of the carpus (wrist)

Hinge joint between humerus and ulna and radius at the elbow

Saddle joint between trapezium of carpus (wrist) and metacarpal of thumb

Pivot joint between proximal ends of radius and ulna

Ball and socket joint between head of the femur and acetabulum of the hipbone

Fig. 3.5 Types of synovial joints (from Salvo SG. Massage therapy: principles and practice. Philadelphia: WB Saunders; 1999).

Obviously, pathological conditions affecting joints will also affect the ROM. Conditions such as contractures, where the soft-tissue components become shortened, will restrict movement, giving rise to hypomobility. This can also occur in situations where the muscle tissue is in a state of spasm. Even fear of pain or discomfort can result in hypomobility. Hypermobility is the opposite pathological condition, and can occur, for example, if the surrounding muscles are weak, or if there has been trauma to the associated tendons, joint capsule or ligaments, and the stability of the joint is adversely affected. Hypermobility in a joint suggests that the structure will be prone to damage caused by excessive ROM.

Some pathological conditions will affect the articulating bones themselves, this will lead to changes in the normal ROM. However, whatever

■ BOX 3.6 Osteoarthritis

This is a common degenerative joint disease, and is caused by 'wear and tear'. It appears to be a natural consequence of the ageing process. It usually affects weight-bearing joints; however, most can be affected, especially those that have been injured. The symptoms are stiffness and pain. Restricted ROM is due to pathological changes, including roughening and erosion of the articulating joint surfaces, the growth of bone spurs on the articulating bones, calcification of the ligaments, thickening of the synovial membrane, and a reduction in the space in the joint cavity. Friction between the joint surfaces is increased, and this causes further degeneration.

the cause of joint dysfunction, surrounding structures will be required to compensate.

MAJOR JOINTS OF THE BODY AND THEIR MOVEMENTS

Joints of the spine

Certain parts of the vertebral column are more mobile than others – notably the areas where one curve joins another – between C7 and T1, T12 and L1, and L5 and S1. These areas are also more prone to injury.

Many of the bodywork therapies are of great value in cases of joint dysfunction, and there are several effective approaches to improving the ROM. For example, massage can decrease muscle spasm, which, in turn, can slightly increase the space in the joint cavity. Massage can also be used to stretch and elongate the connective tissue associated with a joint, helping in some cases to improve mobility. Other modalities and exercises can increase stability of joints, and reduce the risks inherent in hypermobility.

Atlanto-occipital joints

- There are two joints between the atlas and the occiput
- Synovial condyloid joints between the atlas and the condyles of the occipital bone
- Movements – flexion and extension (nodding of the head); lateral flexion.

Atlanto-axial joint

- Synovial pivot joint between the odontoid process of the axis and the facet on the arch of the atlas
- Movements – rotation, shaking of the head.

Intervertebral joints

- Cartilagenous symphyses between the upper and lower aspects of adjacent vertebral bodies
- Intracapsular structure – intervertebral discs
- Movements are limited between individual joints, but over the entire column flexion, extension, lateral flexion and rotation are possible.

Joints of the vertebral arches

- Commonly known as facet joints
- Synovial plane joints between the inferior and superior articular processes of adjacent vertebrae

- Movements – gliding; however, over the entire spine flexion, extension, lateral flexion and rotation movements are possible
- Important strengthening ligaments are the supraspinous ligaments connecting the spinous processes, interspinous ligaments connecting adjacent spines, ligamentum nuchae found in the cervical region connecting the spinous processes and including the occipital protuberance and crest. There are also intertransverse ligaments

■ BOX 3.7 Trauma to vertebrae

Fractures and dislocations are potentially very serious as there is a danger of paraplegia or quadriplegia below the level of the damage.

If the head goes back and then forward very quickly, whiplash may be the consequence. This is dislocation or subluxation in the cervical region. Treatment is usually by traction. Massage is contraindicated.

■ BOX 3.8 Herniated ('slipped') disc

A common cause of low back pain is the condition often referred to as a 'slipped disc'. The *annulus fibrosis* is the outer part of the intervertebral discs, and this can become weak. If the disc is under pressure, e.g. when the spine is flexed and bearing a load, the inner part, the *nucleus pulposus*, can protrude into the adjacent vertebral bodies, and exert pressure on the spinal nerves. This in turn gives rise to a condition known as sciatica. Pain can be severe, protective muscle spasm develops, contributing further to nerve impingement. In severe cases, the disc can rupture.

■ BOX 3.9 Spondylitis, ankylosing spondylitis, spondylosis and spondylolisthesis

These are all pathological conditions affecting the vertebrae and associated structures.

1. *Spondylitis* is a general term used to describe inflamed vertebrae.
2. *Ankylosing spondylitis* is an inflammatory condition, which affects the sacroiliac joints and progresses to affect the intervertebral joints. It is a rheumatoid condition, where the hyaline cartilage is eroded, the bones fuse and ligaments ossify – causing progressive pain and stiffness. The term ankylosis describes complete loss of movement at a joint.
3. *Spondylosis* is the formation of bony spurs at the disc margins of the vertebral bodies. These spurs restrict movement and damage the intervertebral discs.
4. *Spondylolisthesis* is the name given to the condition where one part of a vertebra slips forward over the superior surface of the adjacent vertebra, this usually occurs between the fifth lumbar and the first sacral vertebrae.

Conventional approaches to treating disc degeneration are manipulation, traction and immobilization.

Complementary therapy approaches to these fall mainly in the domain of soft-tissue and movement therapies. Massage, when indicated, can be very effective in the management of back pain due to problems affecting the joints. If structural abnormalities are the cause, or the patient is suffering from inflammatory or degenerative conditions, all of the soft-tissue and movement therapies must be complementary to medical treatment, rather than replacing it, or working in isolation. However, these therapies, if included in a total, holistic treatment programme with other health professionals (such as physiotherapists) are of great benefit to the patient.

connecting the transverse processes and ligamenta flava, which connect adjacent laminae.

Joints of the thorax
Costovertebral joints

The heads of the ribs form synovial plane joints with the facets on adjoining vertebrae.

Costocondral joints

Cartilagenous joints formed by the first seven ribs articulating with the costal cartilage.

Costosternal joints

Fibrous joints formed between costal cartilage and concave depressions on the lateral borders of the sternum.

Joints of the shoulder
The shoulder joint

- Known as the glenohumeral joint
- Synovial ball and socket joint between the head of the humerus and the glenoid cavity of the scapula (Fig. 3.6)
- Bursae are present
- Intracapsular structures include a fibrocartilagenous rim around the glenoid cavity (the glenoidal labrum) and the long head of the biceps muscle

---

■ **BOX 3.10 Dislocation of the shoulder joint**

At the shoulder, a degree of stability has been sacrificed to allow for great mobility. The very shallow glenoid cavity makes the shoulder joint the most mobile of all the joints.

Dislocation is not uncommon – falling on an outstretched hand can result in anterior dislocation. Posterior dislocation may result from direct violence to the anterior part of the shoulder.

Treatment will involve reduction, support and physiotherapy/ rehabilitation exercise.

■ **BOX 3.11 Frozen shoulder**

This chronic condition is more correctly known as adhesive capsulitis – it is a fibrosis of the joint capsule. The causes are not clear, but immobilization/disuse are contributing factors. Conventional treatment approaches are physiotherapy and remedial exercise. Soft-tissue and movement therapies, and aromatherapy are also of benefit, especially with regard to pain relief and elevation of mood.

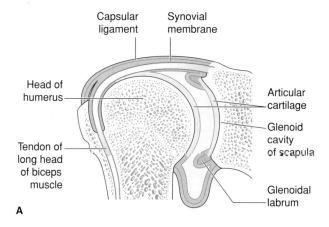

Capsular ligament

Synovial membrane

Head of humerus

Articular cartilage

Glenoid cavity of scapula

Tendon of long head of biceps muscle

Glenoidal labrum

A

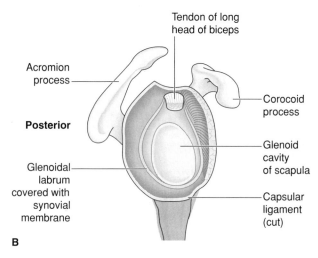

Tendon of long head of biceps

Acromion process

Corocoid process

Posterior

Glenoid cavity of scapula

Glenoidal labrum covered with synovial membrane

Capsular ligament (cut)

B

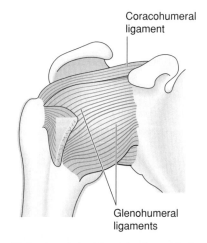

Coracohumeral ligament

Glenohumeral ligaments

C

Fig. 3.6 The shoulder joint. (A) Section viewed from the front; (B) the position of the glenoidal labrum with the humerus removed, viewed from the side; (C) the supporting ligaments viewed from the front. (From Waugh A, Grant A. Ross and Wilson Anatomy and physiology in health and illness. 9th edn. Edinburgh: Churchill Livingstone; 2001.)

- In addition to strengthening ligaments, the capsule is reinforced by the tendons of the 'rotator cuff' muscles
- Movements at the joint are flexion, extension, abduction, adduction, medial and lateral rotation and circumduction.

The sternoclavicular joint

- This synovial gliding joint is formed between the clavicle and the sternum (manubrium)
- In addition to several ligaments, there is a fibrocartilagenous disc within the joint
- Movements follow the movements of the scapula, as no muscles work directly on this joint – elevation, depression, anterior and posterior movement, and rotation are possible.

Acromioclavicular joint

- This is a synovial gliding joint between the clavicle and scapula
- Some individuals do not have this joint
- Movements are anterior and posterior gliding, upward and downward rotation, elevation, depression.

The elbow joint
Ulnarhumeral and radiohumeral joints

- These are synovial hinge joints (Fig. 3.7)
- Movements are flexion and extension
- The olecranon process limits extension.

Radioulnar joint

- This is a synovial pivot joint (Fig. 3.7)
- The interosseous membrane connects the ulna and radius
- Movements are pronation and supination
- During pronation, the radius crosses the ulna into a diagonal position.

The wrist joint
Radiocarpal joint

- The radius articulates with some of the carpal bones – the scaphoid, lunate and triquetrum (Fig. 3.8)
- It is a synovial condyloid joint
- The ulna joins the wrist indirectly by a disc – this allows the movements of pronation and supination without affecting wrist movements
- Movements are flexion, extension and radial and ulnar deviation.

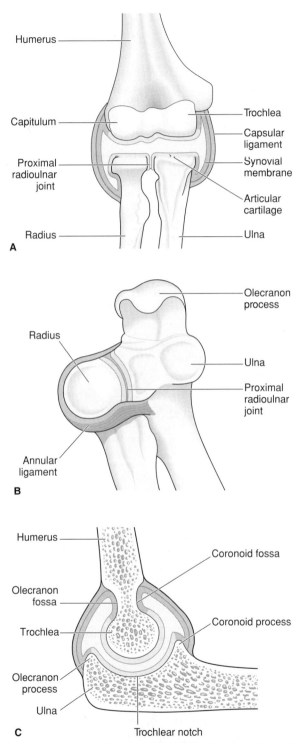

Fig. 3.7 The elbow and proximal radioulnar joints. (A) Section viewed from the front. (B) The proximal radioulnar joint, viewed from above. (C) Section of the elbow joint, partly flexed, viewed from the side. (From Waugh A, Grant A. Ross and Wilson Anatomy and physiology in health and illness. 9th edn. Edinburgh: Churchill Livingstone; 2001.)

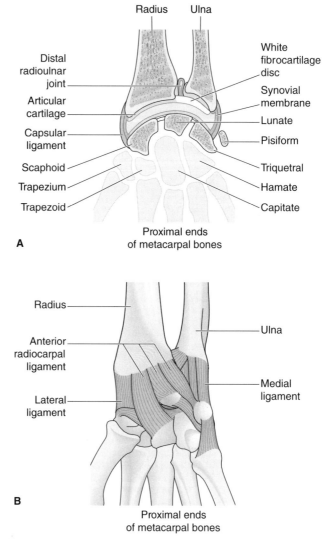

Fig. 3.8 The wrist and distal radioulnar joints. Anterior view. (A) Section; (B) supporting ligaments. (From Waugh A, Grant A. Ross and Wilson Anatomy and physiology in health and illness. 9th edn. Edinburgh: Churchill Livingstone; 2001.)

The hip joint

- The femur articulates in a concave surface, the *acetabulum*, formed by the ilium, pubis and ischium (Fig. 3.9)
- The femoral head is held in place by the *labrum* – a fibrocartilagenous ring around the edge of the acetabulum
- The hip joint is the largest ball and socket joint in the body
- Movements are flexion, extension, abduction, adduction, medial and lateral rotation and circumduction.

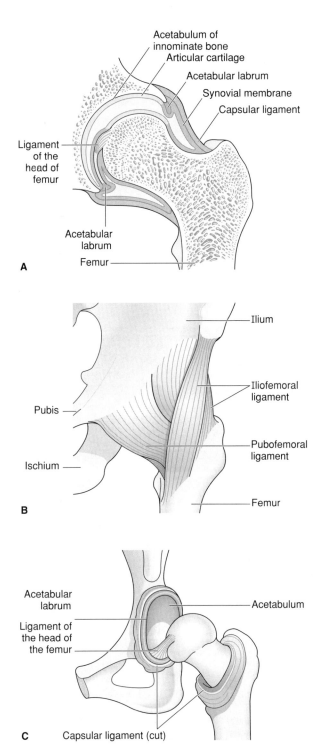

Fig. 3.9 The hip joint. Anterior view. (A) Section; (B) supporting ligaments; (C) head of femur and acetabulum separated to show acetabular labrum and ligament of head of femur. (From Waugh A, Grant A. Ross and Wilson Anatomy and physiology in health and illness. 9th edn. Edinburgh: Churchill Livingstone; 2001.)

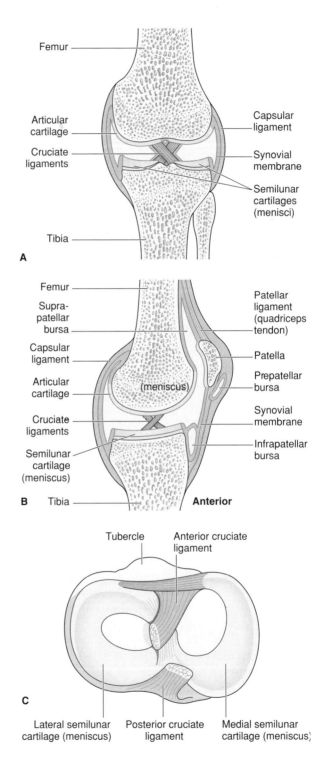

Fig. 3.10 The knee joint. (A) Section viewed from the front. (B) Section viewed from the side. (C) The superior surface of the tibia, showing the semilunar cartilages and the cruciate ligaments. (From Waugh A, Grant A. Ross and Wilson Anatomy and physiology in health and illness. 9th edn. Edinburgh: Churchill Livingstone; 2001.)

The knee joint

- The knee joint is the most complicated joint (Fig. 3.10)
- The articulating bones are the femur and tibia (hinge), and the femur and patella (gliding)
- It is a synovial condylar joint
- Movements are flexion, extension and a degree of medial and lateral rotation when the joint is flexed
- The menisci provide surface contact between the femur and the flat superior surface of the tibia. They act as shock absorbers.
- Important ligaments are the medial and lateral collateral ligaments and the anterior and posterior cruciate ligaments within the capsule.
- The patella moves in the groove between the condyles of the femur. It is important in flexion and extension; it is pulled by the contraction of the quadriceps muscle on the exterior thigh.
- There are several bursae associated with the knee joint.

The ankle joint
Talocrural joint

- The distal ends of the tibia and fibula and the superior surface of the talus form the talocrural (ankle) joint (Fig. 3.11).
- This is a synovial saddle joint, although it is usually classed as a hinge joint
- The main movements are dorsiflexion and plantar flexion; accessory movements in plantar flexion are slight abduction, adduction and rotation
- Important ligaments are the medial collateral (deltoid), lateral collateral and calcaneofibular ligaments.

Inferior tibiofibular joint

This is a fibrous syndesmosis that unites the distal ends of the tibia and fibula, so that they move as one bone at the ankle joint.

The joints of the foot
Intertarsal joints

- These are gliding joints that allow collective movement and weight distribution in the feet
- Movements are limited rotation – eversion and inversion.

Metatarsophalangeal and interphalangeal joints

- These are found in the anterior portion of the feet
- They are hinge joints
- Movements are flexion and extension.

A

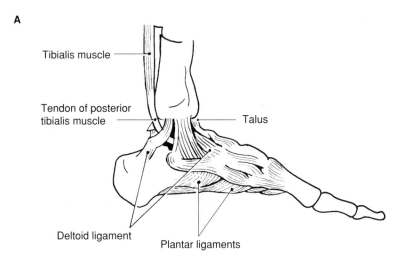

Tibialis muscle

Tendon of posterior
tibialis muscle

Talus

Deltoid ligament

Plantar ligaments

B

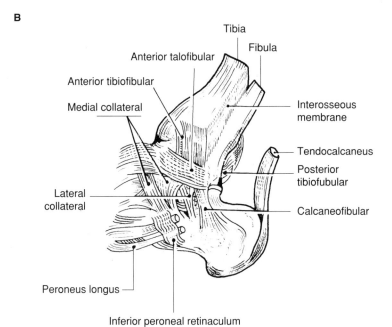

Tibia

Fibula

Anterior talofibular

Anterior tibiofibular

Medial collateral

Interosseous
membrane

Tendocalcaneus

Posterior
tibiofubular

Lateral
collateral

Calcaneofibular

Peroneus longus

Inferior peroneal retinaculum

Fig. 3.11 Left ankle and foot: (A) medial aspect and (B) lateral aspect, to show ligaments (from Bryan GJ. Skeletal anatomy. 3rd edn. Edinburgh: Churchill Livingstone; 1996).

■ BOX 3.12 The arches of the foot

Sprung arches are formed by the bones of the foot, associated ligaments, small muscles in the sole and some tendons of the lower limb Fig. 3.12. The functions of the arches are to transfer body weight without shock and facilitate locomotion – walking, running, jumping.

The *medial longitudinal arch* is highest on the medial aspect of the foot, and is supported by the 'spring' ligament, the plantar ligament, interosseous ligaments and also the tendons of the lower limb.

The *lateral longitudinal arch* is less pronounced and maintained by the short muscles of the foot.

The *transverse arch* runs across the foot, along the bases of the metatarsals.

The reflexologist needs a thorough knowledge of the bones, joints, ligaments and tendons of the foot, in both healthy and abnormal states, in order to be able to locate reflex points with precision and treat with accuracy and sensitivity.

Massage is contraindicated regionally. Complementary therapy approaches to alleviating gout include dietary modifications, and the use of essential oils applied topically in the form of cold compresses for pain relief. As uric acid is a metabolic by-product that is normally excreted in the urine, it is thought that an increased water intake is important in recovery from gout.

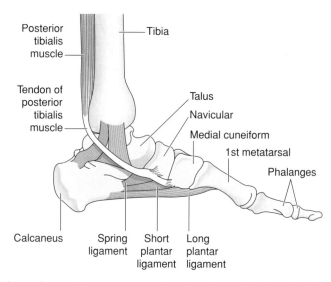

Fig. 3.12 The tendons and ligaments supporting the arches of the foot. Medial view. (From Waugh A, Grant A. Ross and Wilson Anatomy and physiology in health and illness. 9th edn. Edinburgh: Churchill Livingstone; 2001.)

■ BOX 3.13 Gout

Due to metabolic disturbances, excess uric acid in the blood is deposited, as crystals, in the soft-tissue components of the joints. This painful condition is known as gout, and if left untreated, damage to the joint will occur. The most commonly affected joint is the metatarsophalangeal joint of the great toe, and the disease is most common in males over 50 years of age.

THE JOINTS QUESTIONS

Diagrams—Questions 121–124

121–124. A synovial joint

A. Capsule
B. Synovial membrane
C. Ligaments
D. Hyaline cartilage.

121
122
123
124

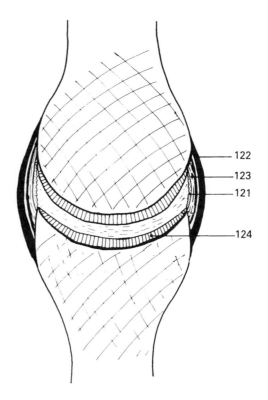

Questions 125–130 are of the multiple choice type

125. Which one of the following statements describes adduction?   125
A. Bending forwards
B. Moving away from the midline
C. Moving towards the midline
D. Turning inwards.

126. The knee joint is a: 126
A. hinge joint
B. gliding joint
C. condylar joint
D. ball and socket joint.

127. Which one of the following is a hinge joint?   127
A. Ankle
B. Metacarpophalangeal joint
C. Temporomandibular joint
D. Wrist.

128. Which one of the following movements is possible at the elbow joint?   128
A. Dorsiflexion
B. Extension
C. Inversion
D. Rotation.

129. The radioulnar joints are: 129
A. gliding joints
B. hinge joints
C. pivot joints
D. saddle joints.

130. The wrist joint is the joint between one of the following groups of bones. Which one?   130
A. The carpus and the metacarpus
B. The distal extremities of the radius and ulna
C. The radius and ulna and the proximal carpal bones
D. The radius and ulna and the distal carpal bones.

Questions 131–136 are of the matching items type

131–133. From the list on the left select the movement that can occur at each joint listed on the right.

A. Plantarflexion	131. Radioulnar joints	131
B. Eversion	132. Tarsal joints	132
C. Supination	133. Wrist joint.	133
D. Ulnar deviation		

134–136. From the list on the left select the anatomical structure which is part of each joint on the right.

A. Acetabulum	134. Knee	134
B. Glenoid cavity	135. Hip	135
C. Lamina	136. Shoulder.	136
D. Obturator foramen		
E. Femoral condyle		

The muscles

4

■ KEY POINTS

- Functions of the muscular system
- Classification of muscle tissue
- Characteristics of muscle tissue
- Skeletal muscle structure
- Muscle contraction
- Coordination of movement
- Muscle names
- The major muscles of the body.

INTRODUCTION

Muscle tissue accounts for between 40 and 50% of the body weight. Muscle tissue is unique in that it can generate force for contraction and movement.

Understanding the muscular system, especially the skeletal muscle system, is essential for all soft-tissue and movement therapists. Therapists who practise massage will require a depth of knowledge that exceeds that of most other disciplines.

Massage has several beneficial effects on the muscular system. Some of these are *mechanical* effects and others are *reflexive* effects elicited via the nervous system. Massage can alleviate tightness, stiffness and spasm, and pain. It improves the blood supply to the muscles – this increases the supply of oxygen and nutrients to the tissues, and also helps the disposal of metabolic waste products. Massage can be used to help resolve dysfunctions of the musculoskeletal system.

CLASSIFICATION OF MUSCLE TISSUE

Three types of muscle tissue are found in the body:

- *skeletal muscle* – the flesh of the body, attached to the skeleton; the muscles that provide locomotion, movement
- *smooth muscle* forms the viscera – for example components of the organs of the digestive, urinary and reproductive systems consist of smooth muscle
- *cardiac muscle* is found only in the heart.

THE FUNCTIONS OF THE MUSCULAR SYSTEM

The functions of the muscular system listed here reflect all three types of muscle tissue.

1. *Movement* – skeletal muscle allows motion and locomotion; it enables us to move our limbs and to move around in our external environment.
2. *Maintenance of body posture* is possible because of skeletal muscle.
3. Skeletal muscle plays a role in the *stabilization of joints*.
4. *Motility* – smooth muscle provides motility, e.g. the movements of the contents of the intestines.
5. *Movement of lymph* is stimulated by contractions of both smooth and skeletal muscle.
6. The *heartbeat* is provided by cardiac muscle.

7. *Generation of heat* – all muscle contractions produce heat. This is vital in homeostasis; the body must be maintained at the correct temperature to function. Shivering occurs if the body becomes cool – this is produced by rapid contractions of skeletal muscle, which generates the heat required.

CHARACTERISTICS OF MUSCLE TISSUE

All muscle tissue is comprised of groups of elongated cells – *muscle fibres*. The microscopic structure, or *histology*, of muscle tissue was introduced in Chapter 1.

All three types of muscle tissue possess the following properties:

- *excitability* – the ability to receive and react to internal and external stimuli
- *contractility* – each muscle fibre can, when stimulated, contract; for this to occur, the muscle must possess a nerve supply and an adequate blood supply
- *extensibility* – the ability to be stretched or extended
- *elasticity* – muscle tissue can return to its original form after contraction or extension.

Smooth muscle tissue

Smooth muscle tissue is classed as *non-striated* muscle tissue as it does not have a striated (striped) appearance when examined under the microscope. It is also referred to as *involuntary* muscle, as this type of muscle is not under conscious control, and as *visceral* muscle, as it is mainly found in the viscera (internal organs).

Smooth muscle tissue contracts in response to nerve impulses, stretching or hormones; its fibres can sustain contraction for fairly long periods, yet the process does not require a great deal of energy. The smooth muscle fibres are each surrounded by a fine membrane, and bundles of these form sheets of muscle tissue. These sheets can form the walls of hollow structures. Thus, smooth muscle tissue is well suited for its locations and functions. For example, it is found in:

- the walls of blood and lymph vessels
- the ducts of exocrine glands
- the organs of the alimentary tract
- the organs of the respiratory tract
- the wall of the bladder
- the wall of the uterus.

Cardiac muscle tissue

Cardiac muscle tissue is only found in the *myocardium*, the wall of the heart. Although it is involuntary, not under the control of the will, striations may be seen when viewed under the microscope. Cardiac muscle cells have a branched appearance. These cellular branches are in very close contact with each other due to *intercalated discs* (microscopic joints), this allows rapid transmission of nervous stimuli throughout the entire myocardium, rather than requiring separate stimulus of discreet bundles of fibres. Thus the contraction of the myocardium is closely coordinated.

Skeletal muscle tissue

Skeletal muscle tissue, unlike smooth or cardiac muscle, is under the control of the will. For this reason, it is often referred to as *voluntary* muscle tissue. It is striated in its microscopic appearance, and is sometimes called striated or striped muscle. There are more than 600 skeletal muscles in the body.

SKELETAL MUSCLE STRUCTURE

Each skeletal muscle could be considered as an individual organ of the musculoskeletal system. Each muscle is composed of thousands of muscle fibres, connective tissue, nerves and blood vessels.

The muscle cell

Muscle fibres are roughly cylindrical in shape, and are generally very long and tapered cells. The horizontal light and dark stripes (striations) seen under the microscope are created by small units called *sarcomeres*. Sarcomeres are the structural units of contraction in muscle fibres.

1. The cell membrane is known as the *sarcolemma*.
2. The cytoplasm of a muscle cell is called the *sarcoplasm*; this contains comparatively large amounts of glycogen (a carbohydrate store which can be converted to an energy source as required) and an oxygen-binding protein called myoglobin.
3. Chains of sarcomeres form *myofibrils*. Myofibrils are packed side by side in the sarcoplasm, forming bundles. Myofibrils consist of thin filaments of *actin* and thicker filaments of *myosin*. These are contractile proteins.
4. Numerous *nuclei* are located just below the sarcolemma.
5. There are many mitochondria, reflecting the energy needs of muscle cells.

Anatomy of skeletal muscle

1. Muscle fibres lie parallel to one another (Fig. 4.1).
2. Each is enclosed within very fine fibrous connective tissue, called *endomysium*.
3. Small bundles of fibres (*fasciculi*) are surrounded by a layer of fascia known as the *perimysium*.
4. These bundles are collectively wrapped in another layer of connective tissue, the *epimysium*. This is fairly tough, and each individual muscle is surrounded by epimysium (Fig. 4.1).
5. This, and the other connective tissues, extend beyond the muscle fibres, enclosing the entire structure, and also extend to become the *tendons*. The point where the muscle ends and the tendon begins is called the *musculotendinous junction*.

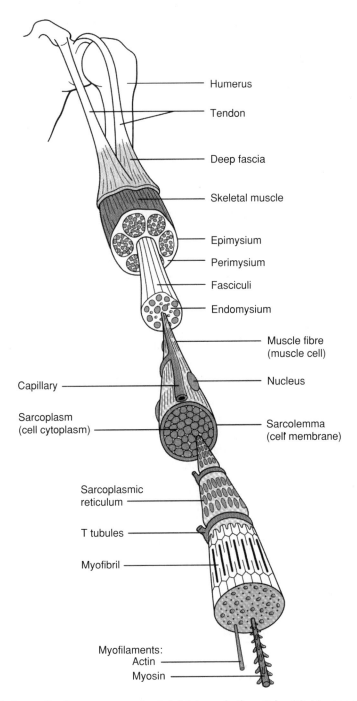

Fig. 4.1 Connective tissue components of skeletal muscle (from Salvo SG. Massage therapy: principles and practice. Philadelphia: WB Saunders; 1999).

Connective tissue components

1. *Tendons* are composed of fibrous connective tissue; they attach muscles to bone, fascia and other soft tissues. They are cord like in appearance.

Some tendons, especially those that cross over joints, have tendon sheaths that are lined with synovial fluid. This serves to reduce friction and protect the tendon. In some cases, *retinacula*, which are retaining bands of connective tissue, may help secure tendons in place. This is found at the knee joints, ankles and wrists.

2. An *aponeurosis* is the name given to a broad, flat, sheet-like tendon.
3. A coarse sheet of fibrous connective tissue surrounds the epimysium. This is the *deep fascia*, it binds the muscles into functional groups. The partitions formed between muscle groups are *intermuscular septa*.

Gross structure of muscle

The shape or form of a skeletal muscle will dictate its possible actions, strength and direction of movement. Muscle shape is determined by the arrangement of the tiny bundles of muscle fibres, the fascicles. There are two basic types of pattern, *parallel* and *penniform*. These are illustrated in Figure 4.2.

1. *Parallel* muscle fibres allow for a great range of motion, but less strength than penniform muscles. They are sometimes called longitudinal muscles. Many of the muscles of the upper limb, where range of movement is important, are of this type.
2. *Penniform* muscle fibres do not afford as much range of movement, but penniform muscles tend to be more powerful. The fibre arrangement resembles a feather. Many muscles of the lower limb, where strength is very important, are of this type.
3. Specialized muscles, called sphincters, are found around external openings to the body. They have *circular* arrangements – the fascicles are arranged in concentric circles, so that when the muscle contracts the sphincter closes.

MUSCLE CONTRACTION

Muscle contraction is stimulated by a nerve impulse, which stimulates the conversion of chemical energy into mechanical energy. Nerves called *motor neurons* stimulate contraction of skeletal muscle. Muscles have specialized receptors for nerve impulses, known as *muscle spindles*. Other types of

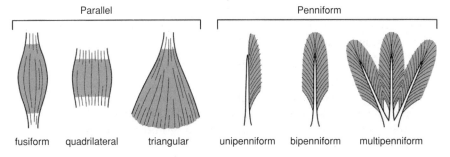

Parallel			Penniform		
fusiform	quadrilateral	triangular	unipenniform	bipenniform	multipenniform

Fig. 4.2 Parallel and penniform muscle fibre arrangement (from Salvo SG. Massage therapy: principles and practice. Philadelphia: WB Saunders; 1999).

> ### ■ Box 4.1 Muscle stress
>
> The main causes of stress to the muscular system, which can lead to dysfunction and diseases are:
>
> - predisposition – inherited factors
> - patterns of use – overuse, misuse, abuse, disuse
> - postural faults
> - emotional stress – highlighting the mind–body link.

receptors are located in tendons (these are known as *tendon organs*), ligaments and joint capsules.

The sliding filament concept

When a skeletal muscle contracts, its individual sarcomeres shorten in length, but the filaments remain unchanged.

Muscle contraction involves thick *myofilaments*, composed of the thread-like contractile protein, *myosin*, and thin myofilaments, composed of *actin*. Together, actin and myosin form chemical cross-bridges with one another. In response to a nervous stimulus, the actin and myosin filaments slide over one another, resulting in simultaneous shortening of all the sarcomeres, and thus the whole cell. A useful analogy is that of sliding doors.

Muscle tone

Even when muscles are relaxed, they must maintain a certain amount of contraction, so that the tissue is ready and able to respond if needed. This is known as *muscle tone*. Muscle tone is controlled by signals from the brain, spinal cord and spindles of the individual muscles. Muscle tone is necessary to maintain good posture and stabilize the joints.

COORDINATION OF MOVEMENT

Muscles do not act independently to produce movement – they work in pairs or groups, called functional units.

Thus for every movement, different muscles within a group assume specific roles (Fig. 4.3). These roles are:

1. *Agonist* – the prime mover, the muscle (or muscles) most responsible for producing the movement.
2. *Antagonist* – the opposing muscle resists or yields to the movement produced by the agonist. It is usually located on the opposite side of the joint. (In the opposite movement, it would become the agonist.)
3. *Synergist* – a muscle (or muscles) that aid the agonist in producing the movement. Synergists are also known as guiding muscles.

4. *Fixator* – a muscle or muscles that support or stabilize the area around the joint, providing a firm base for the movement.

■ **Box 4.2 Muscle damage**

If anything interferes with either the nerve supply or blood supply to a muscle, the muscle will become unable to respond and function normally. For example:

1. An over-tight bandage or plaster cast will interrupt the blood supply, if prolonged the muscle will 'die'.

2. Accidental damage (or disease) of the brain, spinal cord or nerves can result in paralysis.

3. *Spastic paralysis* is a condition where muscles cannot relax – injury or disease of the brain or spinal cord means that the control of the muscles has been cut off. They become contracted and hard, and will pull the affected joints in to abnormal positions.

4. *Muscle spasm* is an increase in muscle contraction, due to excessive motor nerve activity.

5. *Muscle cramp* is a temporary, painful contraction of a muscle or group of muscles – often due to muscle fatigue.

6. If nerves are diseased or damaged, the muscles lose their tone and become *flaccid*, i.e. soft, flabby and unable to contract.

7. *Muscle atrophy* is the decrease in bulk of muscles, a wasting caused by lack of use, damage or disease.

Muscle atrophy can occur very quickly when inactivity is enforced, e.g. bedrest. If possible, active exercises should be encouraged at least every hour. If this is not possible, due to paralysis or unconsciousness, passive movements must be undertaken with the same regularity.

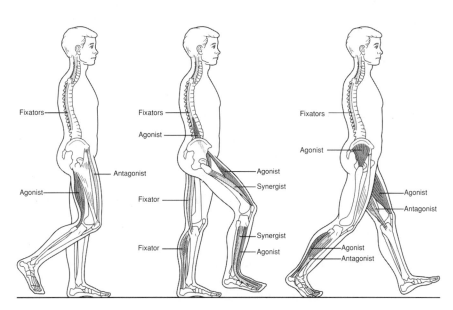

Fig. 4.3 Man walking, depicting agonist, antagonist, synergist and fixators (from Salvo SG. Massage therapy: principles and practice. Philadelphia: WB Saunders; 1999).

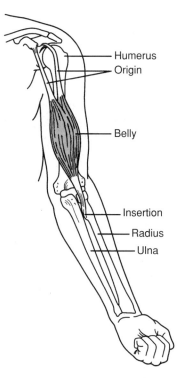

Humerus
Origin

Belly

Insertion
Radius
Ulna

Fig. 4.4 Parts of a skeletal muscle (from Salvo SG. Massage therapy: principles and practice. Philadelphia: WB Saunders; 1999).

ATTACHMENT SITES

Most skeletal muscles consist of a central part, often called the *belly* of the muscle, and two or more points of *attachment*, known as the *origin(s)* and *insertion(s)* (Fig. 4.4):

- the *origin* is usually the proximal attachment site
- the *insertion* is usually the distal point of attachment.

MUSCLE NAMES

It is helpful to understand the meanings of some of the words used to name muscles – the names of muscles often relate to their location relative to the bones, their function, size and shape. For example:

- *sternocleidomastoid* – indicates this muscle's attachments to the sternum, the clavicle and the mastoid process
- *trapezius* – indicates the shape of the muscle; it is a figure with four unequal sides
- *gluteus maximus* and *minimus* – indicates the relative sizes of these muscles
- *frontalis* – indicates the location on the frontal bone
- *levator scapulae* – indicates that the action of the muscle is to raise the scapula

- *extensor hallucis longus* – indicates that the main action of this muscle is to extend the hallux (big toe) and that it is a long muscle.

THE MUSCLES OF THE BODY

It is not the intention of this book to give details of all of the muscles of the body. An *overview* of the main muscles that will be encountered in the practice of soft-tissue and moment therapies, and perhaps in clinical practice, follows (Fig. 4.5).

Muscles of the head face and neck

There are many small muscles in the head, and yet there are only two moveable joints. The muscles that move the temporomandibular joints produce the chewing movements, or mastication. The other muscles of the head are the muscles of facial expression.

1. The muscles of mastication include *temporalis* and *masseter*.
2. The muscles of facial expression include *frontalis*, which raises the eyebrows and wrinkles the forehead, *occipitalis* moves the scalp, *orbicularis oculi* (the winking muscle) produces blinking of the eye, *orbicularis orbis* (the kissing muscle) moves the mouth, *zygomaticus major* (smiling) moves the corners of the mouth, and *buccinator* (mastication, blowing, whistling) compresses the cheeks.
3. The most superficial muscle of the anterior neck is *platysma* – it tightens the skin of the neck and pulls down the lower lip.
4. *Sternocleidomastoid* (SCM) is located on each side of the anterior neck. It is the only muscle that moves the head, which is not attached to any of the vertebrae. The main actions are flexion of the neck and rotation of the head.
5. *Splenius capitus* is a deep muscle of the posterior neck; it extends the head and neck, and also moves the head laterally in a dorsal direction, and rotates it to the side.
6. There are many muscles of the posterior neck; however the major superficial one is *trapezius*. The trapezius covers not only the neck, but also more than half of the back. This muscle is *bilateral*, i.e. it lies on both sides of the spine, and is considered in three parts. The *upper fibres* at the neck produce extension of the head, and elevation and lateral rotation of the scapula; the *middle fibres* retract the scapula; and the *lower fibres* depress and laterally rotate the scapula. This is a muscle of *scapular stabilization*, and the actions depend on whether contraction is unilateral (one-sided) or bilateral.

Muscles that act on the scapula

In addition to trapezius, several other important muscles are classed as muscles of scapular movement and stabilization.

1. *Levator scapula* is a large muscle. Its main action, as its name suggests, is elevation of the scapula, and medial movement of the scapula. However, it can also help stabilize the scapula. Its origins include the

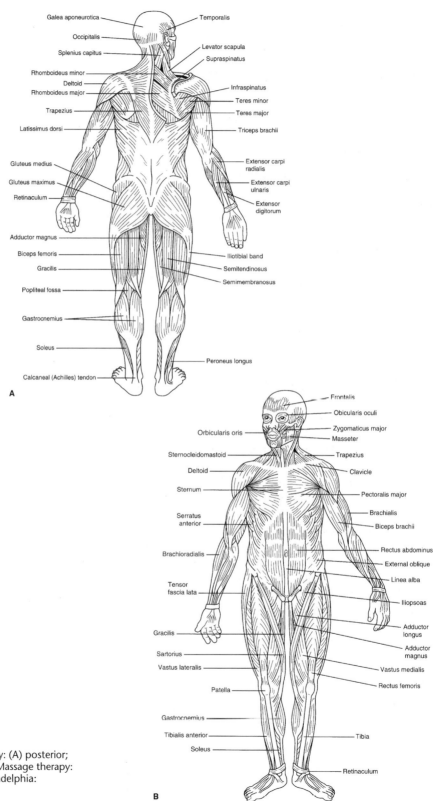

Fig. 4.5 Muscles of the body: (A) posterior; (B) anterior (from Salvo SG. Massage therapy: principles and practice. Philadelphia: WB Saunders; 1999).

atlas and axis, so when the scapula is fixed, it can also produce rotation of the head so that the chin faces the acromion process.

2. *Rhomboideus major* and *minor* (the *rhomboids*) lie under the trapezius. They adduct and elevate the scapula, and rotate it so that the glenoid cavity faces inwards.
3. *Serratus anterior* lies towards the anterior. The name means 'saw like'. Its origins are the first nine ribs, and it produces protraction and lateral rotation of the scapula, in addition to stabilization. It is also an accessory muscle of respiration, as it raises the ribs.

Muscles that act on the shoulder joint

1. *Latissimus dorsi* is the widest muscle of the body – its origins are the spinous processes of T6 to L5, the lower ribs, and the posterior superior iliac crest and the sacrum. It inserts at the bicipital groove of the humerus. Latissimus dorsi extends, medially rotates and adducts the shoulder. Although its actions are at the shoulder, it is often the cause of back pain if its lower attachments are damaged.
2. *Teres major* is a synergist to latissimus dorsi and it adducts the arm. The name *teres* means smooth and round.
3. *Supraspinatus, infraspinatus, teres minor* and *subscapularis* are collectively known as the *rotator cuff muscles*. They originate on the scapula, cross the shoulder joint; their tendons converge and merge with the fibrous capsule of the shoulder joint. They are sometimes called 'lively ligaments' – their main function is to secure the head of the humerus in the glenoid cavity and to reinforce the joint capsule. They all produce movement at the shoulder joint and arm, including adduction and rotation movements. Subscapularis is often implicated in the condition known as 'frozen shoulder'.
4. The *deltoid* is the muscle that provides the characteristic rounded contour of the shoulder. The name comes from the Greek *delta*, which means triangular. It is comprised of three sets of fibres – posterior, middle and anterior – each producing different movements, including flexion, extension, abduction and medial and lateral rotation of the arm.
5. *Pectoralis major* forms the upper part of the anterior chest. It adducts and medially rotates the arm, and also assists in elevating the thorax if the arm is in abduction.

Muscles of the upper limb

These can be considered in three groups: the muscles that act on the elbow, wrist and hand joints.

Muscles that act on the elbow joint include:

- *biceps brachii* – which flexes the shoulder and the elbow, and supinates the forearm
- *triceps brachii* – which extends the shoulder and the elbow
- *brachioradialis* – located on the radial side of the forearm, is an elbow flexor
- *pronator teres* lies across the anterior surface of the elbow joint, it is an elbow flexor, but also produces pronation of the forearm, as its name indicates

- *supinator* supinates the forearm, and can also assist in elbow flexion when the hand is halfway between pronation and supination.

The bellies of muscles that act on the hand are located in the forearm, and taper to long tendinous insertions in the hands. The tendons, enclosed in tendon sheaths, are secured at the wrists by flexor and extensor retinacula. Generally, the muscles on the anterior of the forearm/wrist are *flexors*, while the muscles on the posterior are the *extensors* of the wrist and hand.

1. *Flexor carpi radialis, palmaris longus* and *flexor carpi ulnaris* are the flexors in the anterior superficial layer.
2. *Extensor carpi radialis longus* and *brevis, extensor digitorum, extensor digiti minimi, extensor carpi ulnaris* and *extensor pollicis brevis* are the extensors in the posterior superficial layer.

There are a few very small muscles on the hands – these are known as *intrinsic muscles*. They are located on the *thenar eminence* (the pad below the thumb on the palmar surface) and the *hypothenar eminence* (the pad below the little finger on the palmar surface). There are also a few deep muscles. The musculature of the human hand is unique – it allows for a huge range of fine movements.

Muscles of the hip region

The muscles that form the gluteals (buttocks) are the most powerful in the body:

- *gluteus maximus* extends the hip on the thigh
- *gluteus medius* and *minimus* abduct and medially rotate the thigh.

Other muscles that act on the hip joint are:

- *iliopsoas,* – the principal flexor of the hip joint
- *deep lateral rotators* are located beneath the gluteals; the largest is the *piriformis.*

Muscles of the thigh region

Here, muscles may act on the hip or knee, or, in some cases, both joints. *Lateral* muscles include:

- *tensor fascia lata* – located on the lateral aspect of the hip and thigh; its action is the same as the gluteus medius and minimus – hip abduction, flexion and medial rotation. It assists knee extension, as it inserts at the iliotibial band.

The main *posterior* thigh muscles are the *hamstrings* – three muscles that collectively *extend the hip and flex the knee*:

- *biceps femoris* is the more lateral muscle of the group
- *semimembranosus* is the medial hamstring
- *semitendinosus* lies over semimembranosus.

In the *medial* part of the thigh, the main action of the muscles is *adduction of the thigh* on the hip. Muscles here include:

- *gracilis* (this is also involved in knee flexion)
- *adductor magnus*, *adductor longus* and *adductor brevis*.

The principal group of muscles on the *anterior* thigh is *quadriceps femoris*. This group of four muscles shares a common insertion at the tibial tuberosity – thus the common tendon of these muscles crosses the knee joint. The main action of the 'quads' is *extension of the knee*. The 'quads' are:

- *rectus femoris* – which originates at the anterior inferior iliac spine, thus flexes the thigh on the hip joint as well as extension of the knee
- *vastus intermedius* – which lies under rectus femoris
- *vastus medialis*
- *vastus lateralis*.

The other significant muscle of the anterior thigh is:

- *sartorius* – known as the 'tailor's muscle' because in times gone by, tailors sat in a cross-legged position. Sartorius is the longest muscle in the body; it crosses over the hip and knee joints, passing over quadriceps femoris. The actions are lateral rotation and flexion of the hip, and flexion (and assists medial rotation) of the knee – all requirements for sitting in a cross-legged position.

Muscles of the lower leg

Muscles of the lower leg act at the knee joint, ankle joint and foot. They can be considered in three compartments – a deep fascial sheath separates each compartment. The muscles of the anterior compartment are extensors (dorsiflexors). Dorsiflexors are very important in walking; they prevent the toes from dragging. The muscles of the lateral compartment produce eversion and plantar flexion, and the muscles of the posterior aspect assist knee flexion and produce plantar flexion and inversion of the foot.

Muscles of the *anterior compartment* are:

- *tibialis anterior* – which is located over the lateral shaft of the tibia; its actions are dorsiflexion and inversion of the foot
- *extensor digitorum longus* – which is located over the fibula and inserts at the distal phalanges; it produces dorsiflexion and also extension of the toes (excluding the big toe).
- *extensor hallucis longus* – inserts at the distal phalanx of the big toe; it produces extension of the big toe and assists dorsiflexion.

Muscles of the *lateral compartment* are:

- *peroneus longus* and *brevis* – produce eversion and assist plantar flexion.

The main muscles of the *posterior compartment* are the following.

1. *Gastrocnemius*, this is the bulky, fleshy muscle of the lower leg. It has two *heads* (attachment points, which are superior to the medial and lateral epicondyles of the femur), two fleshy fusiform bellies, and a common insertion at the calcaneus via the *Achilles tendon*. It is a

bi-articular muscle – it acts on two joints – assisting knee flexion and producing plantar flexion.

2. *Soleus*, which lies behind gastrocnemius; it is named after the flat, sole fish that it is thought to resemble. It shares insertion with gastrocnemius via the Achilles tendon, and produces plantar flexion.

3. *Tibialis posterior* is an elongated, thin muscle located over the posterior tibia and inserting at the plantar aspect of some of the foot bones. It assists plantar flexion and produces inversion.

4. *Flexor digitorum longus* (FDL) is responsible for flexion of the toes (excluding the big toe); it also supports the longitudinal arch when standing.

5. *Flexor hallucis longus* flexes the big toe, and like FDL it supports the longitudinal arch of the foot.

Muscles of the trunk and vertebral column

The deep (intrinsic) muscles of the vertebral column produce movements of the trunk, but are also important in stabilization, posture and maintaining the curves of the spine. These muscles are organized in groups that work in a coordinated fashion, allowing a wide range of movements in various regions of the spine. These movements include extension, hyperextension, flexion, lateral bending and rotation.

The group known as the *paraspinals* extends from the occiput to the sacrum, and includes:

• the *erector spinae* group (sacrospinalis) – termed vertical muscles; their principal actions are extension, rotation and lateral flexion of the vertebral column
• the *transversospinalis* group – oblique muscles that lie deep to the erector spinae.

The *abdominal muscles* and extensive fascia form the anterior abdominal wall. In addition to producing movement, these muscles have an important role in functions such as defecation, urination and breathing. They are also involved in coughing and laughing. The fibres of the abdominal muscles run in four directions; this arrangement produces a criss-cross network that provides firm support for the internal organs, and allows compression of the abdomen. The abdominals are also important in posture, especially of the lumbar region.

The abdominals attach to the *linea alba* – a strong fibrous band of connective tissue that extends from the xiphoid process to the symphysis pubis. The group comprises the following.

1. *Rectus abdominus* – produces flexion of the trunk and compression of the abdomen; also lateral flexion of the vertebral column. This muscle extends from the costal cartilage of the ribs and the xiphoid process to the symphysis pubis – its length is maintained by four bands of connective tissue (tendinous intersections) running across the muscle at intervals.

2. *External* and *internal abdominus oblique* – produce flexion of the trunk, lateral flexion of the vertebral column and compression of the abdomen.

3. *Transverse abdominus* – compresses the abdomen.
4. *Quadratus lumborum* – does not act on the abdominal contents, but produces tilting of the pelvis in a forward direction and hyperextension of the spine; also lateral flexion of the trunk and elevation of the hip.

The muscles of the pelvic floor

The levator ani and the coccygeus muscles form the pelvic floor.

1. The *levator ani* are flat muscles attached to the pelvis. They unite with each other forming the pelvic floor, which supports the pelvic organs. There are three openings through the *female pelvic floor*. The anterior opening is the *urethral orifice*, leading from the bladder. The middle opening, the *vaginal orifice*, leads to the uterus, the posterior opening forms the *anus*, the exit from the bowel. The male pelvic floor has only the urethral and anal openings. The area between the anus and the anterior openings is the *perineum*. Weakness in the perineum can result in prolapse of the pelvic organs.
2. The *coccygeus* supports the coccyx and assists in closing the posterior part of the pelvic outlet.

The muscles of the thorax

The thoracic muscles are the *intercostal* muscles and the *diaphragm* – they produce the movements that allow breathing. Three layers of muscles form a wall around the front and sides of the thorax, and the diaphragm forms the muscular partition between the thoracic and abdominal cavities.
   The intercostal muscles lie between the ribs:

- the *internal intercostals* depress the rib cage – this moves air out of the lungs when exhaling
- the *external intercostals* elevate the rib cage – this increases the size of the thoracic cavity and draws air into the lungs when inhaling.

The *diaphragm* is important in the process of breathing in. When relaxed, it is a dome-shaped sheet of muscle that is attached to the lower ribs, the first three lumbar vertebrae and the xiphoid process. The muscle fibres arch upwards and converge inwards to form a central tendon of insertion – this is an *aponeurosis*. When the diaphragm contracts, it pulls and flattens the central tendon, the belly of the muscle flattens out and this expands the thoracic cavity.

THE MUSCLES QUESTIONS

Diagrams—Questions 137–149

137–140. The muscles of the body (posterior)

A. Biceps femoris
B. Trapezius
C. Deltoid
D. Gastrocnemius.

137
138
139
140

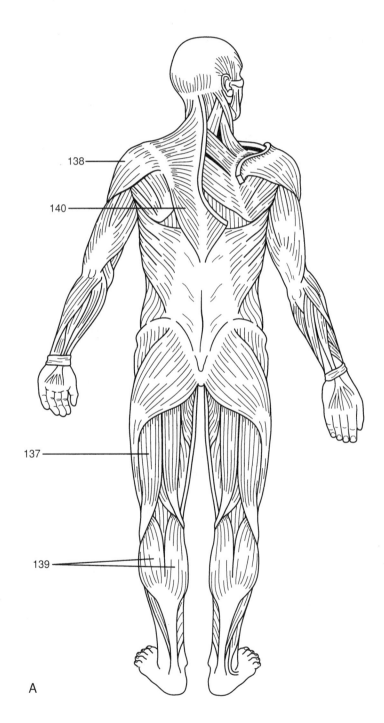

A

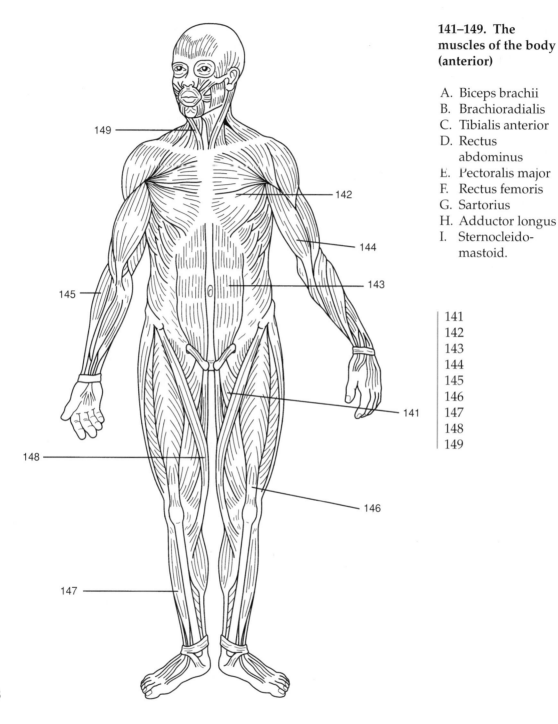

141–149. The muscles of the body (anterior)

A. Biceps brachii
B. Brachioradialis
C. Tibialis anterior
D. Rectus abdominus
E. Pectoralis major
F. Rectus femoris
G. Sartorius
H. Adductor longus
I. Sternocleido-mastoid.

141
142
143
144
145
146
147
148
149

B

Question 150–151 are of the multiple choice type

150. Which one of the following is a waste product of muscle contraction?   150
  A. Carbon monoxide
  B. Glucose
  C. Oxygen
  D. Water.

151. Paralysis is the condition which results from: 151
  A. Dead muscle tissue
  B. Diseased muscle tissue
  C. Muscle deprived of its nerve supply
  D. Muscle deprived of its blood supply.

Questions 152–171 are of the true/false type   **T** | **F**

152–155. A muscle fibre:
    152. is its cell
    153. is striped longitudinally
    154. has more than one nucleus
    155. is the covering of the muscle.

156–159. The diaphragm:
    156. is a dome-shaped muscle
    157. is a muscle of respiration
    158. rises when it contracts
    159. separates the thorax from the abdomen.

160–163. The deltoid muscle:
    160. lies over the shoulder joint
    161. adducts the upper limb
    162. raises the shoulder girdle
    163. connects the upper limb to the shoulder girdle.

164–167. The gluteal muscles:
    164. cover the sciatic nerve
    165. flex the hip
    166. keep the trunk upright in walking
    167. rotate the hip.

168–171. Quadriceps femoris:
    168. extends the hip
    169. extends the knee
    170. is the medial muscle of the thigh
    171. is inserted into the tibia.

Questions 172–174 are of the matching items type

172–174. From the list on the left select a movement which is produced by each muscle listed on the right.

A. Abduction of the shoulder	172. Intercostals	172
B. Extension of the neck	173. Sternocleidomastoid	173
C. Rotation of the head	174. Trapezius.	174
D. Mastication		
E. Inspiration		

The circulatory system

5

■ KEY POINTS

- The heart
- The blood vessels
- The structure of the blood vessels
- The circulation of the blood
- The blood

- The lymphatic system
- A summary of the circulation
- Blood pressure
- The cardiac cycle
- The pulse.

INTRODUCTION

The circulatory system consists of the heart, the blood vessels and the blood. It is the means by which nutrients and oxygen are conveyed from the digestive tract and lungs to the body cells. The waste products are also conveyed by this system from the cells to the organs that excrete them. The heart acts as a pump, keeping the blood circulating through the blood vessels.

Some harmful substances, which are dangerous if present in the body, enter a secondary circulation called the lymphatic system, where they may be destroyed before reaching the bloodstream. This system consists of lymphatic vessels, nodes and ducts. A clear yellowish fluid called lymph circulates through these vessels. The spleen, an abdominal organ, is also associated with this system.

The circulatory and lymphatic systems communicate with each other and will be studied together.

THE HEART

The heart is a hollow, cone-shaped, muscular organ which lies between the lungs in the space in the middle of the thorax called the *mediastinum* (see Fig. 1.7). It is tilted slightly more towards the left side than to the right. It is situated behind the sternum and in front of the oesophagus and the large blood vessels. The base of the heart lies uppermost to the right side of the chest at the level of the second rib. The apex is on the left side in contact with the diaphragm at the level of the fifth and sixth ribs.

The outside of the heart is covered by fibrous tissue and the inside is lined with epithelium. The epithelial tissue forms valves which divide the organ into two upper and two lower chambers. The chambers are called the *atria* (upper) and the *ventricles* (lower). The right and left atria are uppermost at the base of the heart and the right and left ventricles are below at the apex. The blood flows from the atria to the ventricles from where it is pumped round the body and lungs.

The pericardium

The outer covering of the heart is called the pericardium. It is a sac of fibrous tissue lined with another double-layered sac of epithelial tissue. The outer fibrous sac is continous with the covering of the large blood vessels which enter and leave the heart at its base. It is protective in function and, because it is tough, it prevents the heart from overdistending. The inner sac has two layers. The outermost layer is called the *parietal pericardium* and lines the fibrous sac. The inner layer, the *visceral pericardium*, is adherent to the heart muscle itself. Between these two layers is a potential space filled with a very small amount of serous fluid which allows for smooth movement between the two layers when the heart beats.

The myocardium

The wall of the heart is made of cardiac muscle tissue and is called the myocardium. This tissue also forms a *septum*, dividing the organ into a right and left side. Cardiac muscle tissue is specialized, found only in the heart, and all of the individual cells are in very close contact with each other so it resembles a 'sheet' of tissue. It is not under control of the will. It is stimulated to contract by small areas of specialized tissue dispersed in the wall – the so-called *pacemaker* of the heart.

The myocardium is thinner in the atria which receive blood from the blood vessels, and thicker in the ventricles which push the blood out into the lungs and the general circulation. The function of the myocardium is to act as a pump. It contracts and squeezes the blood out, and when it relaxes it allows the heart to fill up with blood again.

The endocardium

The endocardium is made of squamous epithelium and forms a smooth lining for the blood to flow over. It is continuous with the lining of the blood vessels. The smooth surface prevents clots forming in the blood.

Double folds of endocardium with some fibrous tissue form the valves which divide the atria from the ventricles and prevent the blood flowing in the wrong direction. The *atrio-ventricular valve* on the right side has three flaps or cusps and is sometimes called the *tricuspid valve*. The left atrio-ventricular valve has two cusps and is sometimes known as the *bicuspid* or *mitral valve* (Fig. 5.1).

These valves open and close with the flow of the blood. They are attached to the ventricle walls by fibrous cords (*chordae tendineae*) which prevent the valves from turning inside out.

THE BLOOD VESSELS

There are three types of blood vessels:

- arteries, which carry blood away from the heart
- capillaries, which connect the arteries to the veins
- veins, which return the blood to the heart.

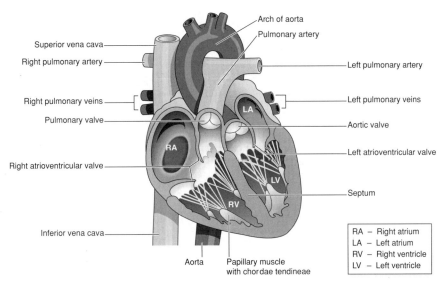

Fig. 5.1 (from Waugh A, Grant A. Ross and Wilson Anatomy and physiology in health and illness. 9th edn. Edinburgh: Churchill Livingstone; 2001).

■ **BOX 5.1 Valvular disease**

In endocarditis or valvular disease of the heart, the valves may leak or the opening may become so small that insufficient blood gets through. The result of valvular disease is a slowing down of the circulation and an accumulation of excess fluid in the tissues and in the lungs. This excess fluid in the tissue results in the swelling (oedema) of the ankles and the breathlessness that often accompany this disease.

The arteries

The arteries leave the heart at the right and left ventricles, where they are very large. They branch again and again, getting smaller and thinner and spreading out to every part of the body. The smallest arteries are called *arterioles*. Eventually, these vessels become so small they cannot be seen without a microscope. The arterioles have now become capillaries.

The capillaries

The capillaries are minute vessels which form a network throughout the tissues. They eventually join up to form small veins called *venules*.

The veins

The venules join other venules until veins are formed (Fig. 5.2). The largest veins enter the heart at the right and left atria.

THE STRUCTURE OF THE BLOOD VESSELS

The arteries and veins are constructed in a similar way to the heart. They are muscular tubes with a protective covering and a smooth lining. The

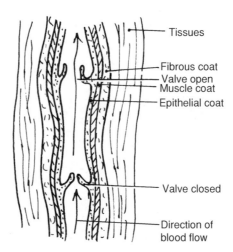

Fig. 5.2 Longitudinal section of a vein.

muscle coat (*tunica media*) is involuntary muscle tissue which is supplied by nerves from the autonomic system (see Ch. 10). This tissue can contract and relax, varying the size of the vessel, depending on the amount of blood required by the tissue it supplies. The muscular walls also contain elastic tissue which allows the vessel to stretch and recoil, depending on the amount of blood it contains. There is more elastic tissue in the large arteries than in the small arteries, and there is very little in the veins (Fig. 5.3). The veins have much thinner and softer walls than the arteries: they collapse when cut. Blood will flow from cut veins, but it spurts from cut arteries, which retain their shape.

The fibrous covering of the vessels (*tunica adventitia*) is protective in function. The epithelial lining (*tunica intima*) is continuous with the endocardium. It forms valves in the large veins of the limbs where it prevents backflow of the blood as it travels up against gravity. Valves are also present where the large arteries leave the heart.

The walls of the capillaries are continuous with the lining of the arterioles and the venules. They are composed of a single layer of epithelial cells which is thin enough to allow water and nutrients to pass through from the

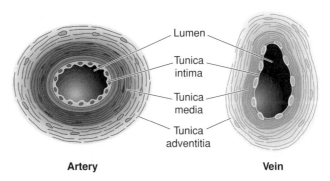

Fig. 5.3 (from Waugh A, Grant A. Ross and Wilson Anatomy and physiology in health and illness. 9th edn. Edinburgh: Churchill Livingstone; 2001).

■ BOX 5.2 Arteriosclerosis aneurysm and infarct

Arteriosclerosis is a hardening or narrowing of the muscular wall of an artery, limiting the flow of blood to the part it supplies. This is often the lower limb and can cause severe pain on walking. The pain is due to oxygen starvation of the tissues.

An aneurysm is a weak part in the vessel wall which dilates and may burst, causing severe haemorrhage.

An infarct is an area of dead tissue. This is often the result of a blocked artery which prevents oxygen from reaching the tissues. When arterial blockage occurs in the myocardium, it causes death of part of the heart muscle (cardiac infarct) and may result in cardiac arrest.

blood to the tissue fluid. The capillaries form a vast network in all the tissues of the body.

THE CIRCULATION OF THE BLOOD

When we talk about the circulation we mean the passage of the blood from the heart via the arteries to the capillaries and back to the heart via the veins (Fig. 5.4). We will be considering the circulation as separate systems but, of course, each system communicates with the others.

The coronary circulation

The heart itself is the first organ to receive a blood supply. Two important arteries branch from the aorta just as it leaves the left ventricle. These are

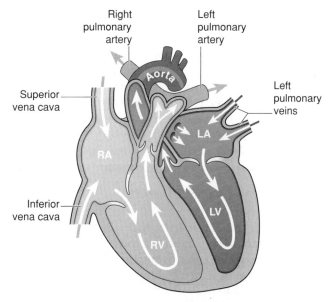

Fig. 5.4 Blood flow through the heart (from Waugh A, Grant A. Ross and Wilson Anatomy and physiology in health and illness. 9th edn. Edinburgh: Churchill Livingstone; 2001).

■ **BOX 5.3 Coronary thrombosis**

A coronary thrombosis is the sudden blocking of a coronary artery by a clot. This is a common cause of sudden death or myocardial infarction. If the blockage is incomplete, the patient may suffer from severe pain in the region of the heart and down the left arm. This condition is called angina pectoris.

the *coronary* arteries. These arteries divide and become arterioles and then capillaries. The capillaries join to form venules and veins. The coronary veins drain into a channel called the *coronary sinus* which lies in the wall of the right atrium, the chamber which receives the venous blood. This system of blood vessels is called the coronary circulation and is the means by which the wall of the heart is nourished.

The general or systemic circulation

The general circulation consists of the arteries and veins which carry the blood from the left ventricle round the body and back to the right atrium.

The aorta

The blood leaving the left ventricle of the heart passes through the aortic valve into the *aorta*. This is the largest artery in the body. The aorta passes upwards then arches over the base of the heart to lie at the back. It passes down through the thorax posteriorly, through an opening in the diaphragm where it enters the abdomen.

The circulation to the upper limbs

Leaving the arch of the aorta, where it lies at the base of the neck, are two *subclavian* arteries. These pass into the *axillae* and down the upper arm where they are renamed the *brachial* arteries. The brachial artery divides in front of the elbow to form the *radial* and *ulnar* arteries. These lie in the lateral and medial sides of the forearm and enter the hand by passing over the wrist. In the hand they become the *palmar* and *digital* arteries.

The blood returns from the hand by the veins which lie beside the arteries, sharing their names. The *subclavian* veins join with the veins of the head to form the *brachio-cephalic* veins. These in turn join to form the superior vena cava which enters the right atrium (Fig. 5.5).

The circulation to the head and neck

The right and left common carotid arteries which lie in the neck are branches of the arch of the aorta. These arteries divide and become the *internal* and *external carotid* arteries. The internal carotid arteries enter the skull and supply the brain. The external carotids divide to supply the face and scalp. Two of their branches can be felt pulsating; the *temporal* in front of the ears and the *facial* arteries in front of the angles of the jaw.

Blood returns from the head and neck by the *jugular* veins which join up with the right and left subclavian veins (see Fig. 5.6).

Massage strokes that involve pressure are applied in the direction of the heart or thorax. This can assist venous circulation. Massage can only directly affect superficial and peripheral circulation.

The radial artery can be felt pulsating at the base of the thumb, where it lies on top of the radius. This is the most common site for feeling the pulse. Any change in rate, force or rhythm of the pulse should be detected and reported.

The brachial artery is the one that, in First Aid, can be compressed against the humerus to arrest bleeding following an injury to the forearm or hand.

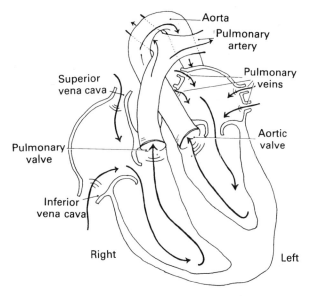

Fig. 5.5 The blood vessels of the heart.

The circulation in the thorax

The thoracic aorta is the part of the aorta which lies behind the heart. This large artery gives off branches which supply the chest wall, part of the lungs and the oesophagus. Blood from these parts is returned to the heart by veins which join the *superior vena cava*.

The circulation in the abdomen

The abdominal aorta is the continuation of the thoracic aorta which passes through the back of the diaphragm and continues down through the abdomen. It lies in front of the vertebrae, to the level of the fourth lumbar vertebra, where it divides to form the right and left *common iliac* arteries. The abdominal aorta provides branches to the abdominal organs. There are two *phrenic* arteries which supply blood to the diaphragm, the *renal* arteries which supply the kidneys, and the *ovarian* and *testicular* arteries which supply the reproductive organs.

Single arteries supply the other organs. The *hepatic* and *splenic* arteries go to the liver and the spleen respectively. The *gastric* artery supplies the stomach, and the *superior* and *inferior mesenteric* arteries carry the blood supply to the bowel.

Veins from the reproductive organs, the kidneys, the liver and the diaphragm enter the *inferior vena cava*. This large vein is formed by the junction of the two common iliac veins which bring blood from the lower limbs. This vein lies at the back of the abdomen to the right of the aorta. It passes through the centre of the diaphragm and enters the heart at the right atrium.

The circulation to the lower limbs

The common iliac arteries divide in the pelvis to form the *internal* and *external iliac* arteries. The internal iliac arteries supply the pelvic organs.

■ **BOX 5.4 Varicose veins**

Varicosed veins have defective valves. As a result, the return of venous blood to the heart is sluggish, the veins dilate and the legs become swollen and painful. The skin nutrition of the legs is impaired and leg ulcers may develop. Varicose ulcers are very slow to heal.

The external iliac arteries pass out of the pelvis into the thighs where they change their names to the *femoral* arteries.

The femoral artery passes round to the back of the knee to become the *popliteal* artery. This artery divides to form the *anterior* and *posterior tibial* arteries which supply the leg and become the *plantar* and *digital* arteries of the foot.

The veins in the lower limbs lie alongside the arteries and have the same names. These are called the deep veins. There is, however, a second set of veins lying just under the skin. These *superficial* veins join the deep vein at the knee and in the groin. They are not supported by surrounding muscles and may become varicosed.

The pulmonary circulation

An important group of vessels carries venous blood containing excess carbon dioxide from the heart to the lungs. In the lungs the carbon dioxide is excreted by expiration and the blood becomes reoxygenated before being returned to the heart and then into the systemic circulation (see Ch. 6).

The pulmonary artery leaves the right ventricle and divides into two branches, one to each lung. Blood is returned to the left atrium by the four pulmonary veins, two from each lung (see Fig. 5.5). This is one of the few places in the body where an artery carries deoxygenated blood and a vein carries oxygenated blood.

The portal circulation

The portal circulation carries blood containing nutrients from the stomach, spleen and bowel to the liver (see Ch. 7). The gastric vein, the splenic vein and the mesenteric veins all unite to form the large portal vein which enters the liver.

THE BLOOD

Blood is a very active tissue. It carries nutrients, oxygen, hormones, waste products and antibodies from one organ to another. It connects the different parts of the body and is therefore described as a connective tissue. It has a fluid matrix in which cells float. The average individual has about 5–6 litres of circulating blood.

Everyone knows that blood is a warm, red, sticky and salty fluid. If blood is withdrawn from an individual's vein and is allowed to stand in a test-tube, the red part falls to the bottom and a clear yellowish fluid is left above.

The blood is now divided into a solid part and a fluid part. The fluid part is called *plasma* and the solid part consists of the cells or *blood corpuscles*.

The plasma

About 55% of the blood volume is plasma. This is mainly water with certain substances dissolved in it, some of which come from the food that we digest.

1. *Nutrients*:
   a. glucose from carbohydrate foods such as potatoes and sugar
   b. amino acids from protein foods such as meat and fish;
   c. fats from such foods as milk and butter
   d. vitamins from all foods.
2. *Mineral salts*: These have many uses and help to maintain the slight alkalinity of the blood. Examples are sodium chloride and sodium bicarbonate, as well as small amounts of potassium, calcium, magnesium, phosphates, copper and iron.
3. *Waste products*: these are mainly carbon dioxide and urea.
4. *Plasma proteins*: albumin, which exerts an osmotic force and makes the blood sticky.
5. *Clotting substances*: these are prothrombin and fibrinogen.
6. *Antibodies*
7. *Hormones*: These are secretions of the endocrine glands.

The blood cells

There are three types of blood cells:

- red blood corpuscles or *erythrocytes*
- white blood corpuscles or *leucocytes*
- platelets or *thrombocytes*.

Erythrocytes

These cells give the blood its colour. They make up about 99% of the total number of blood cells. They are usually described as biconcave, non-nucleated, distensible discs. There are about 5 million in one cubic millimetre of blood in men, and slightly fewer in women. They tend to adhere to each other and, under the microscope, appear as piles of cells. These erythrocytes can squeeze through the finest capillary. Each cell contains *haemoglobin*, a substance that has an affinity for oxygen. When the erythrocytes reach the capillaries that surround the air sacs in the lungs, the haemoglobin combines with oxygen and transports it to all the tissue cells. Erythrocytes carrying oxygen (forming *oxyhaemoglobin*) are bright red, but when they have given the oxygen up to the cells they become bluish red in colour. The blood in the arteries is, therefore, bright red and in the veins it is bluish. Haemoglobin is an iron-containing protein.

Erythrocytes are developed in the red bone marrow. Mature erythrocytes cannot develop unless *vitamin B_{12}* is present. When they reach maturity they pass into the bloodstream where they convey oxygen to the tissue cells. This oxygen-carrying function of the erythrocytes is of vital importance. Each red cell lives for approximately 4 months. It is then destroyed

■ BOX 5.5 Vitamin B$_{12}$

Vitamin B$_{12}$ (cyanocobalamin) is found in certain foods. Before it can be absorbed, a substance secreted by the stomach, called the *intrinsic factor*, must be present. If this factor is absent, the red blood cells do not develop properly and the individual suffers from *pernicious anaemia*.

■ BOX 5.6 Anaemia

Anaemia means a deficiency of haemoglobin. This may be due to a lack of red blood cells or to a deficiency in their haemoglobin content. The most common type of anaemia is *iron-deficiency* anaemia, which may be due to a loss of blood or to a lack of iron in the diet.

Some complementary therapies, including massage therapies, reflexology and aromatherapy, are said to strengthen the immune system. They may support immune function by aiding homeostatic mechanisms. It has been shown that the numbers of white blood cells and the numbers of natural killer cells increase following massage – this may support the claim.

Some of the essential oils used in aromatherapy have *cytophylactic* properties – they increase the activity of leucocytes in the defence of the body against infection.

by the spleen and broken down into its component parts. The iron is recycled and used by the bone marrow to manufacture more haemoglobin. The protein part is carried to the liver where it forms one of the ingredients of bile. As cells die they are replaced. If many cells are lost, as in the case of haemorrhage, then the red bone marrow produces more.

Leucocytes

The white blood corpuscles are the scavengers of the body. They have what is called a phagocytic action. They travel to an area of tissue which has become infected by microorganisms, surround the organisms, destroy and digest them. They can be compared to an army going abroad to fight the enemy. However, if the organisms are virulent, the result can be destruction of the affected tissue and the cells. This is how *pus* is formed. It consists of dead tissue cells, leucocytes and microorganisms.

Several different types of *leucocyte* are formed in the bone marrow. They are larger than the erythrocytes, much fewer in number and all possess a nucleus. Some of the leucocytes have very fine granules in the protoplasm and are called *granulocytes*. Granulocytes can squeeze through the capillary wall to attack invading microorganisms. Others have no granules and are called *agranulocytes*. These are subdivided into *lymphocytes* and *monocytes*. Lymphocytes are to be found in the blood, the *tonsils*, the *spleen* and the *lymph nodes*. These corpuscles destroy microorganisms and play a part in the formation of antibodies. *Antibodies* destroy any substance which is foreign to the body. These foreign substances are called *antigens*. The presence of an antigen stimulates the production of more lymphocytes. Some monocytes circulate in the bloodstream and are phagocytic. Some migrate into tissues where they develop into macrophages. They also have a role in inflammation and immunity.

When organ transplantation is undertaken, the body recognizes the presence of foreign material. Drugs must be given to suppress the action of the leucocytes so that the new organ will not be rejected by the body. Anyone given these immunosuppressive drugs must be protected from exposure to infection.

Thrombocytes

These are small oval discs present in the blood in large numbers. They do not possess a nucleus and are smaller than the other cells. They also come from the bone marrow.

Thrombocytes are sticky. When the wall of a blood vessel is damaged they stick together and *plug up the hole until* a clot is formed.

■ BOX 5.7 Leukaemia

Leukaemia is a malignant disease affecting the white blood cells. They increase in number, are immature and crowd out the healthy cells. An acute type of leukaemia occurs in children and, if untreated, is quickly fatal.

The clotting mechanism The thrombocytes liberate a substance called thromboplastin which acts on the *prothrombin* and *calcium* in the blood producing *thrombin*. Thrombin acts on the *fibrinogen* in the plasma and *fibrin* is formed. The threads of fibrin form a network in which the blood cells are trapped. This is the clot which will occlude the opening in the blood vessel and prevent bleeding (see Table 5.1).

If you study the formation of a clot in a test-tube you will see that it shrinks, and as it does so a clear, yellowish fluid appears. This is serum and it consists of plasma minus the clotting substances.

■ BOX 5.8 Thrombus, embolus

A *thrombus* is a clot forming in an intact vessel. It is commonly caused by a narrowing of, or damage to, the blood vessel wall. This is usually accompanied by a sluggish circulation. The presence of a thrombus in the deep veins of the calf is a relatively common complication of bedrest. This is one of the reasons why early ambulation and leg exercises should follow surgery whenever possible.

An *embolus* is a solid body or an air bubble carried in the circulation. Part of a thrombus may become detached and travel in the bloodstream to the heart, where it may block the pulmonary artery. This is a pulmonary embolism; it is a complication of deep venous thrombosis and can be rapidly fatal.

Blood groups

When blood transfusion is required a specimen of blood is sent to the haematology department to be grouped and crossmatched. Before blood is transfused it must be checked very carefully to ensure that blood is received which is compatible. Blood must be of the correct group.

In the walls of the red blood corpuscles there are antigens, and in the plasma, antibodies. Remember that antibodies destroy antigens. The

Table 5.1 The mechanism of clotting

Thrombocytes		Blood plasma		
Thromboplastin	+	Calcium and prothrombin	=	Thrombin
Thrombin	+	Fibrinogen	=	Fibrin
Fibrin	+	Blood cells	=	Clot

Thromboplastin is also known as Factor III, and prothrombin as Factor II.

antigens are called *agglutinogens* and are classified A, B, AB or O. The antibodies are called *agglutinins* and are classified Anti-A and Anti-B.

Individuals are divided into four blood groups A, B, AB and O. If a person's blood belongs to group A, his antigen is A but his antibody is Anti-B. If he is transfused with blood group B which contains Anti-A antibodies the donor cells will clump together (agglutinate). This blood is incompatible and the patient will become very ill. His temperature will rise, he may become jaundiced and the clumped cells may block the kidney tubules, causing renal failure.

An individual with blood group AB has no agglutinins (antibodies) and can therefore receive blood from any other group. He is known as a universal recipient.

An individual with blood group O has Anti-A and Anti-B agglutinins (antibodies) but no agglutinogens (antigens). There are, therefore, no antigens to be destroyed so he can give his blood to any group. This person is a universal donor.

Crossmatching means taking some of the donor cells together with the recipient's plasma and observing if clumping of the cells occurs (see Table 5.2).

The rhesus factor

In the blood of three-quarters of the world population there is a substance called the rhesus factor. Those of us who have this factor are said to be rhesus positive, the others are rhesus negative. Normally, there are no antibodies in the plasma against the rhesus factor, but if rhesus-positive blood is given to a rhesus-negative patient, rhesus-positive antibodies will appear in the blood. Any subsequent transfusion of rhesus-positive blood might be fatal, as the patient now has antibodies which will act against the transfused cells.

A pregnant woman who is rhesus negative may be carrying a child who has inherited rhesus-positive blood from its father. A reaction may occur in the blood of this fetus, causing destruction of the red cells and jaundice. To prevent severe damage it is sometimes necessary to change the child's blood completely either before or after birth.

THE LYMPHATIC SYSTEM

The lymphatic system consists of an additional set of vessels through which some of the tissue fluid passes before reaching the large veins and

Table 5.2		
Cell-antigen	*Group* **Plasma-antibody**	*Transfusion* **Can be transfused with**
A	Anti-B	A and O
B	Anti-A	B and O
AB	None	A, B, AB and O
O	Anti-A and Anti-B	O

entering the blood (Fig. 5.6). This system consists of *lymphatic capillaries, vessels, ducts* and *nodes*. The fluid in the system is called *lymph*.

Lymphatic capillaries are present in many tissues. They form networks in the tissue spaces but, unlike the blood capillaries, they start as blind tubes with rounded ends. They are larger than the blood capillaries and more porous, allowing such substances as microorganisms to pass from the tissue fluid to the lymph (see Fig. 5.7).

The lymphatic vessels are similar in structure to the small veins. They have more valves and these give them a beaded appearance. Several vessels enter one lymphatic node, but the lymph leaves the node by one larger vessel. Eventually, the larger vessels join up to form ducts which are about the size of medium-sized veins. There are two lymphatic ducts. The *thoracic duct* commences below the diaphragm, passes into the thorax and joins the systemic circulation in the neck at the junction of the left subclavian and jugular veins. The right lymphatic duct is only about 1 cm in

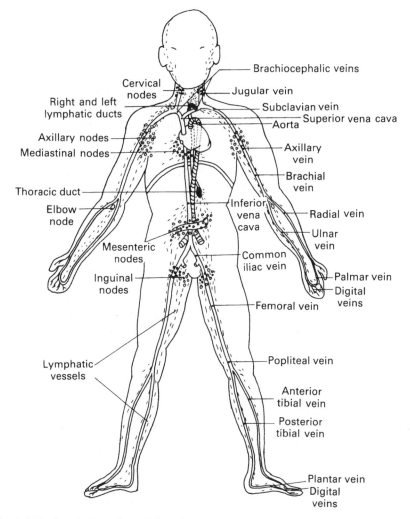

Fig. 5.6 The lymphatic nodes and the veins.

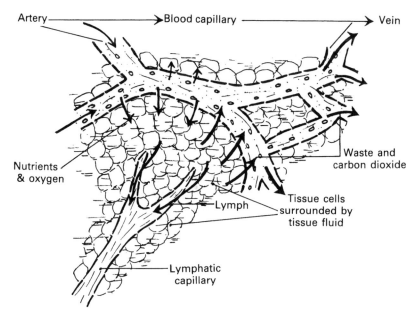

Fig. 5.7 The movement of tissue fluid.

length and opens into the junction of the right subclavian and the right jugular veins.

The lymphatic nodes are generally about the size and shape of small beans and are situated at strategic points in the body. They contain lymphocytes and the lymph must pass through one or more of these nodes before it enters the bloodstream. The nodes act as filters, preventing the passage into the blood of any bacteria, damaged cells or tumour cells which may have passed from damaged tissue into the lymph. The lymphocytes break down these substances but, unfortunately, are not always able to hold back invading organisms or tumour cells.

Infection from a sore throat may result in swollen painful 'glands' in the neck, which can be palpated easily. These so-called glands are the *cervical lymph nodes* which filter the lymph from the head and neck. A septic finger may cause swelling of the *axillary nodes*, and if lymphatic vessels are inflamed a red streak can be seen on the arm. A septic toe can cause swelling of the *inguinal nodes* which are situated in the groin.

There are lymphatic nodes in the *thorax, abdomen* and *pelvis*. These nodes are closely related to the organ they drain. The nodes receiving lymph from the intestines are situated in the *mesentery* which is the covering of the intestines. These nodes become enlarged in infection and tumours of the bowel. The lymphatic drainage of the chest is into the nodes which lie in the *mediastinum*, the space between the lungs in which the heart lies. In city dwellers and cigarette smokers the lymph in these nodes is often black from inhaled dirt and smoke.

The tonsils

There are several other areas of lymphoid tissue in the body. The tonsils form part of a protective ring of tissue at the entrance to the respiratory and digestive tracts. Lymphatic vessels leave the tonsils and enter the cervical nodes.

The spleen

The spleen is a purplish, half-moon-shaped organ in the left hypochondriac region of the abdomen. It lies below the diaphragm and behind the lower ribs, and is mainly composed of lymphoid tissue enclosed in an elastic fibrous capsule.

The spleen has several functions. It contains lymphocytes, some of which get into the bloodstream to carry out their phagocytic action. It destroys worn out erythrocytes, producing bile pigments and iron. It produces antibodies and is capable of providing extra red blood corpuscles in cases of emergency when there is hypoxia. Hypoxia means that there is a diminished amount of oxygen in the tissues. The extra erythrocytes increase the amount of oxygen that can be carried in the blood.

The spleen can only be felt if it is enlarged. Enlargement may occur in a variety of conditions. One of these is acute infection, when the spleen enlarges to meet the increased needs of the body for lymphocytes. The spleen can be removed surgically with few serious effects on the patient, as other tissues in the body take over its functions.

The thymus gland

The thymus gland is a soft, greyish-pink gland which is present in the thorax behind the sternum. It is large in infants and growing children and it reaches its maximum size at puberty. After puberty this gland gradually disappears until in adult life there is only a minute piece of fatty tissue left.

The functions of the thymus are not completely understood, but it is necessary for the development of lymphoid tissue in infancy.

A SUMMARY OF THE CIRCULATION

Having studied the structure and function of the various parts of the circulatory system, we will now consider the work of the circulation as a whole.

The system is full of blood. There are about 5–6 litres in the normal individual. The heart beats once every four-fifths of a second, that is about 75 times per minute. The pumping action is stimulated by electrical impulses from the pacemaker (*sinoatrial node*) in the wall of the right atrium. The atria contract and push the blood through the atrio-ventricular valves into the ventricles. The electrical signals now reach the ventricles through the *atrio-ventricular node* and the atrio-ventricular bundle (*bundle of His*). This tissue carries the electrical impulses to the walls of the ventricles, causing them to contract. The contraction pushes the blood out into the systemic and pulmonary circulations by the aorta and the pulmonary artery. At this stage the atrio-ventricular valves are closed and the aorta and pulmonary valves are open. The muscular walls of the atria and the ventricles then relax and the heart fills up with blood once more.

Venous blood enters the right atrium through the inferior and superior venae cavae and arterial blood enters the left atrium by the four pulmonary veins. This is the only part of the circulation where venous blood flows through arteries and arterial blood flows through veins. The blood containing carbon dioxide leaves the right ventricle by the pulmonary artery and travels to the lungs where the interchange of gases takes place. The oxygenated blood then returns to the left atrium by the four pulmonary veins.

The septum of the heart not only divides it into two sides but it separates the arterial blood from the venous blood.

The blood leaves the heart by the large arteries, which have elastic walls. As the blood is pushed into them these arteries stretch, and when the heart relaxes they recoil. This pushes the blood along into the smaller vessels. Eventually, this arterial blood reaches a network of capillaries. At the arteriole end of this network, water, oxygen and nutrients are pushed through the walls of the capillaries into the tissue fluid by the pressure of the blood. The tissue fluid circulates through the tissues, giving up oxygen and nutrients to the cells and collecting waste products (Fig. 5.7).

There are two routes by which the water and waste can get back into the bloodstream. Some of the fluid is sucked through the walls of the capillaries at the venule end by the osmotic force of the albumin in the blood. The rest returns to the blood, having gone through the lymphatic system. If there is an abnormality of the lymphatic vessels or insufficient albumin in the blood, fluid will collect in the tissues. The part becomes swollen and will 'pit' if pressed by the fingers. This condition is called *oedema*.

The blood in the capillaries and the lymph in the lymphatic capillaries must now get back to the heart by the veins and lymphatic vessels. As the heart dilates between each contraction, venous blood is sucked into the right atrium. This is assisted by the action of the diaphragm in deep breathing. Inspiration has a sucking effect on the blood in the inferior vena cava and on the lymph in the thoracic duct. The muscles in the limbs have a similar sucking effect on the veins and lymphatic vessels. When they contract they 'milk' the blood and lymph up towards the heart. The numerous valves prevent back-flow. Gravity plays an important part in returning the blood to the heart from the head and neck, and also from the upper limbs when they are held above the shoulders.

Massage can reduce oedema by improving lymphatic circulation. A specialized technique known as *manual lymphatic drainage* can be used in clinical situations to reduce lymphoedema.

There are lymph capillary plexuses on the soles of the feet. The rhythmical compression movements of reflexology can improve lymphatic circulation.

BLOOD PRESSURE

Blood pressure is the pressure exerted by the blood on the walls of the blood vessels. Blood pressure is equal to the cardiac output times the resistance against the vessel walls (total peripheral resistance). The pressure in the large arteries varies as the heart contracts and relaxes. The maximum pressure is exerted upon the artery walls when the heart contracts and is known as the systolic pressure. The diastolic pressure is the force exerted upon the vessel walls when the heart is relaxing. Blood pressure varies from person to person. Age, gender and other variables influence blood pressure. Normal pressures are said to range between 100 and 150 mmHg systolic and from 60 to 90 mmHg diastolic.

Therapeutic massage can temporarily reduce the blood pressure.

There are thus several factors which, working together, maintain the blood pressure within normal limits. These are:

- the amount of blood circulating (blood volume)
- the force with which the heart pumps (cardiac output)
- the elasticity of the large arteries
- the calibre of the small arterioles (peripheral resistance).

The amount of blood circulating

This will be less in shock and haemorrhage. A badly injured patient or a patient who has had a major operation will have a low blood pressure if untreated. If blood has been lost, as in haemorrhage, this is replaced by whole blood. If the blood volume has been reduced, as in some forms of shock, saline or dextrose solution may be given until the volume of the blood circulating has been returned to normal.

The cardiac output

This depends on the volume of blood which returns to the heart by the veins. If the venous return is poor, the amount of blood leaving the heart is less. Less force is required, the heart beat is weak and the blood pressure is low. If we have to stand still for long periods of time, the venous return from the lower limbs is inhibited because of gravity and lack of exercise. The heart beat weakens and the blood pressure falls, which sometimes results in a faint.

The elasticity of the large arteries

This maintains the continuous flow of the blood out to the periphery of the body. As they stretch and recoil they push the blood into the smaller vessels. If the walls of the vessels are hardened, as they may be in old age, the pressure of the blood against the inelastic walls is greater.

The peripheral resistance

This is the state of slight contraction of the muscular walls of the arterioles, producing resistance to the flow of blood. These vessel walls can dilate or contract, depending on the amount of blood required by the organ they supply. Heat causes *vasodilation* in the skin and cold causes *vasoconstriction*. When the vessels are dilated the pressure is lower and when they are constricted the pressure is greater.

A badly shocked patient has a low blood pressure. This fall in pressure is compensated for by constriction of the arterioles in the skin. This is why the patient's skin looks white and feels cold. It is dangerous to overheat the patient because this will cause vasodilation which will make the skin feel warmer but the heat will lower the blood pressure still further.

THE CARDIAC CYCLE

Blood pressure is recorded by a *sphygmomanometer*. There are always two recordings, one low and the other high. The higher pressure is normally around 110 millimetres of mercury (110 mmHg) and is the pressure in the arteries when the heart is contracted. This period of contraction is called

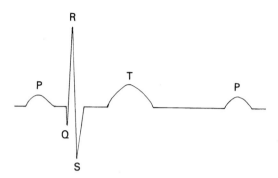

Fig. 5.8 Cardiac cycle.

systole. Systole lasts for two-fifths of a second. The pressure recorded is called the *systolic* blood pressure. The contraction is followed by a period of rest when the heart fills up with blood. This period also lasts for two-fifths of a second and is called *diastole*. During diastole the heart is not pumping and the pressure is less, usually about 80 mmHg. This is *diastolic* blood pressure. Blood pressure is recorded with the systolic pressure noted above and the diastolic pressure noted below (110/80 mmHg).

The *cardiac cycle* consists of *systole* plus *diastole* and takes place every four-fifths of a second. The other fifth is the beginning of the next cycle. The cycle therefore occurs about 70 times each minute.

The beat of the heart is controlled by electrical impulses from the pacemaker. This electrical activity can be recorded on an *electrocardiograph*. The tracing of one cardiac cycle will appear as shown in Figure 5.8.

The P wave is the period of contraction of the atria, Q, R and S is the contraction of the ventricles and T is the beginning of the period of rest.

A stethoscope is used to listen to the heart beat. This is placed over the apex of the heart and the heart sounds will be heard. These are described as 'lubb dup' and are the sounds made by the valves closing.

THE PULSE

The pulse is the beat of the heart as felt at an artery. The pulsation is caused by the stretching of the elastic walls of the arteries during systole when the heart is pushing blood out into the aorta. This wave of distension extends out to the periphery and can be felt where an artery lies over bone. By counting the pulsations, a record can be made of the rate at which the heart is beating. At the same time, various other pieces of information about the heart and blood vessels can be obtained.

The pulse may be rapid or slow, weak or strong, rhythmical or irregular. These observations will tell you about the state of the heart. A rapid, weak pulse may be a sign of internal haemorrhage. The heart beat is weak because the volume of blood going into it is less. It is rapid in order to get the reduced volume of blood round the body. An irregularity in rhythm denotes an irregular heart beat. The time between each beat should be the same but sometimes one beat may be much weaker than others and appears to be 'missed'.

The normal pulse rate changes with the position of the individual. It is quicker when an individual is active and slower when he is at rest. A child has a more rapid pulse than an adult and a woman's pulse is more rapid that a man's. Emotion and exercise increase the pulse rate. A trained athlete, however, has a slow pulse but a much stronger heart beat.

THE CIRCULATORY SYSTEM QUESTIONS

Diagrams—Questions 175–195

175–181. The heart

A. Left atrium
B. Aorta
C. Pulmonary artery
D. Pulmonary veins
E. Inferior vena cava
F. Left atrio-ventricular valve
G. Pulmonary valve

175
176
177
178
179
180
181

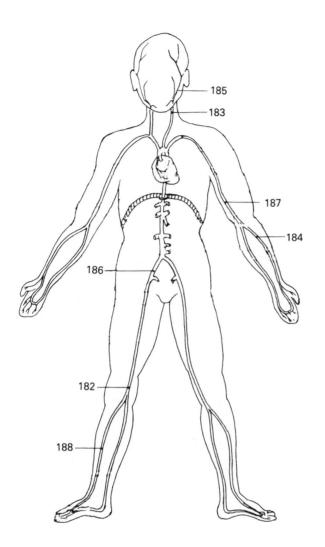

182–188. The arteries

A. Carotid
B. Radial
C. Brachial
D. Facial
E. Common iliac
F. Anterior tibial
G. Popliteal

182
183
184
185
186
187
188

189–195. The veins and lymphatic vessels

A. Jugular vein
B. Axillary nodes
C. Mesenteric nodes
D. Inguinal nodes
E. Thoracic duct
F. Mediastinal nodes
G. Cervical nodes

| 189 |
| 190 |
| 191 |
| 192 |
| 193 |
| 194 |
| 195 |

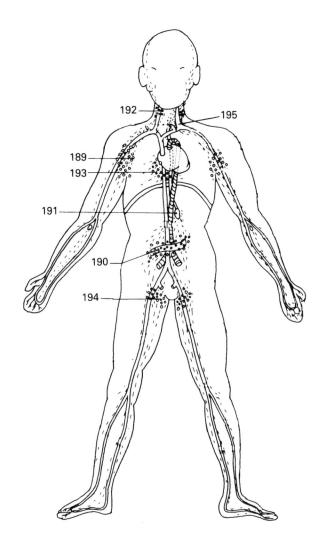

Questions 196–205 are of the multiple choice type

196. The total volume of blood in the average body is: 196
  A. 3–4 litres
  B. 5–6 litres
  C. 7–8 litres
  D. 9–10 litres.

197. The blood is: 197
  A. slightly acid
  B. slightly alkaline
  C. neutral
  D. strongly alkaline.

198. Which of the following is the most accurate definition of anaemia?   198
  A. Bloodlessness
  B. Deficiency of haemoglobin
  C. Deficiency of iron
  D. Deficiency of cyanocobalamin.

199. Which of the following arteries is not a direct branch of the abdominal aorta?   199
  A. Phrenic
  B. Renal
  C. Internal iliac
  D. Mesenteric.

200. Which one of the following veins does not enter the inferior vena cava?   200
  A. Gastric
  B. Ovarian
  C. Renal
  D. Phrenic.

201. Which one of the following statements is true?   201
  A. Lymphatic capillaries are less permeable than blood capillaries
  B. Lymphatic nodes are similar to glands with ducts
  C. Lymphatic vessels contain numerous valves
  D. The thoracic duct lies entirely within the thorax.

202. Which one of the following statements is true? Blood travels from: 202
  A. The left atrium to the aorta
  B. The left ventrical to the vena cava
  C. The right ventricle to the pulmonary artery
  D. The right atrium to the pulmonary veins.

203. Which one of the following is not a factor which maintains the blood pressure?   203
  A. The volume of blood in the blood vessels
  B. The pressure of valves in the veins
  C. The cardiac output
  D. The peripheral resistance.

204. The cardiac cycle normally occurs once in: 204
   A. 1 second
   B. 0.1 second
   C. 0.3 second
   D. 0.8 second.

205. Which one of the following will slow the rate of the heart?   205
   A. Emotion
   B. Exercise
   C. Physical training
   D. Haemorrhage.

Questions 206–253 are of the true/false type   T | F

206–209. The heart
    206. lies in front of the oesophagus
    207. lies behind the bronchus
    208. lies with its apex in contact with the diaphragm
    209. lies with its base tilted towards the left.

210–213. The coronary sinus
    210. is a cavity in the skull
    211. is part of the nerve supply to the heart
    212. is to be found in the right atrium
    213. contains venous blood.

214–217. The inferior vena cava
    214. is formed by the junction of the common iliac veins
    215. enters the right atrium
    216. passes through the diaphragm
    217. lies to the left of the aorta.

218–221. Erythrocytes
    218. have a phagocytic action
    219. synthesize haemoglobin
    220. transport oxygen
    221. are greater in number in women than in men.

222–225. The spleen
    222. is essential for life
    223. can produce extra erythrocytes in an emergency
    224. destroys erythrocytes
    225. contains lymphocytes.

226–229. Diastole is part of the cardiac cycle. During diastole:
    226. the atria and ventricles are relaxed
    227. the atrio-ventricular valves are closed
    228. the blood is entering the heart by the pulmonary veins
    229. the blood pressure is increased.

230–233. If a blood transfusion is necessary, a person who belongs to group:
    230. O can give blood to group A
    231. AB can receive blood from group A
    232. B can receive blood from group AB
    233. A can give blood to group B.

234–237. A thrombus:
    234. is a clot formation in a blood vessel
    235. is common in the veins of the leg
    236. is the same as an embolus
    237. is a relatively common complication of bedrest.

238–241. The blood pressure: T | F
    238. falls in shock
    239. falls in immobility in the upright position
    240. rises in cold conditions
    241. falls in old age.

242–245. Venous blood returns to the heart by:
    242. contraction of the heart
    243. gravity
    244. the sucking action of the diaphragm
    245. the 'milking' action of the muscles.

246–249. When the skin arterioles constrict:
    246. heat is lost from the body
    247. the blood pressure rises
    248. the pulse rate increases
    249. the skin becomes pale.

250–253. Osmotic pressure is the force that:
    250. draws tissue fluid through the walls of the capillaries into the blood
    251. pushes the fluid from the blood to the tissue cells
    252. returns the blood to the heart
    253. sends blood into the general circulation.

Questions 254–265 are of the matching items type

254–256. From the list on the left select the tissue which forms each part of the wall of the heart listed on the right.

A. Areolar tissue	254. Endocardium	254
B. Cardiac muscle tissue	255. Myocardium	255
C. Fibrous tissue	256. Pericardium.	256
D. Squamous epithelium		
E. Voluntary muscle tissue		

257–259. From the list on the left select the tissue which forms each part of the wall of the arteries on the right.

A. Areolar tissue	257. Tunica adventitia	257
B. Cardiac muscle tissue	258. Tunica intima	258
C. Elastic fibrous tissue	259. Tunica media.	259
D. Squamous epithelium		
E. Involuntary muscle tissue		

260–262. From the list on the left select the statement which describes the cells on the right.

A. Help in the clotting of blood	260. Erythrocytes	260
B. Contain fibrinogen	261. Leucocytes	261
C. Help in the formation of antibodies	262. Thrombocytes.	262
D. Contain calcium		
E. Contain iron		

263–265. From the list on the left select the substance present in the plasma which is best described by each word on the right.

A. Albumin	263. Mineral	263
B. Enzyme	264. Protein	264
C. Glycerol	265. Waste.	265
D. Potassium		
E. Urea		

The respiratory system

6

INTRODUCTION

All of the cells of the body require a constant supply of energy to enable them to operate. This energy is mainly obtained from chemical reactions which can only take place in the presence of oxygen, obtained from the atmosphere (Table 6.1). Carbon dioxide is produced during these reactions as the main waste product and must be got rid of from the body.

The exchange of oxygen for carbon dioxide is called respiration and it is the function of the respiratory system. Transport of gases from the lungs to the air is by a series of passages. These passages allow the air containing the vital oxygen to enter the lungs and come in close contact with the blood. This part of respiration is called inspiration. Inspiration is followed by expiration and then a pause.

On inspiration, the blood takes up oxygen from the air. On expiration, air containing less oxygen and more carbon dioxide is breathed out. Most of the carbon dioxide has been carried in the blood plasma to the lungs in the form of *carbonic acid* or *sodium bicarbonate*.

The interchange of gases between the air in the lungs and the blood is called *external respiration*. *Internal respiration* refers to the diffusion of oxygen from the capillaries into the extracellular fluid surrounding the cell and then into the cell itself. Carbon dioxide diffuses from the cell, through the extracellular fluid and then into the capillary. Diffusion of these gases is from an area of high concentration to one of a low concentration, i.e. down the concentration gradient.

The organs of the respiratory system are the air passages and the lungs. The air passages consist of the nose, the pharynx, the larynx, the trachea and the bronchi. The lungs consist of the bronchi, the bronchioles and the

Table 6.1 Composition of the atmosphere

Inspired air		Expired air	
Oxygen	20%	Oxygen	16%
Carbon dioxide	0.04%	Carbon dioxide	4.04%
Nitrogen	78%	Nitrogen	78%
Other inert gases	1%	Other inert gases	1%
Water vapour	variable	Water vapour	saturated

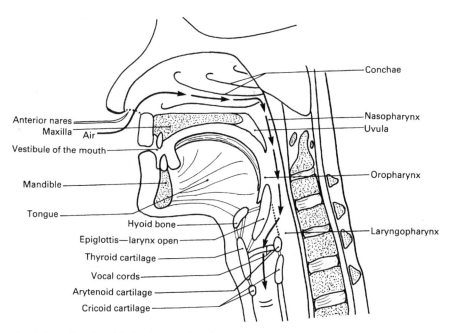

Fig. 6.1 Section through the head and neck.

air sacs or alveoli. Because the nose and the larynx are parts of the air passages, two related functions of the respiratory system are smell (see Ch. 11) and speech.

THE AIR PASSAGES

The nose

The nose consists of two parts: the external nose and the nasal cavity.

The external nose protrudes from the face and has a skeleton which is composed of cartilage in its lower part. The upper part, or bridge of the nose, consists of the two *nasal* bones.

The nasal cavity is a large cavity in the skull which is divided into two parts by a septum. Projecting from the walls of this cavity are the upper, middle and lower *conchae* (turbinate bones) (Fig. 6.1). These are scroll shaped bones under which are the openings into the nasal sinuses. The septum and the conchae greatly increase the surface area of the nasal cavity. This increase in surface area means that there is a corresponding increase in the lining tissue of the nose which consists of ciliated columnar epithelium (mucous membrane), continuous with the mucous membrane lining the sinuses and the nasal part of the pharynx. This membrane has an important function.

As air is breathed in through the nostrils (the anterior nares), it comes in contact with the mucous membrane. The mucus makes the lining moist and sticky, and it is warm because it has a rich blood supply. The air, therefore, is warmed and moistened. As the mucus is sticky, particles of dust, bacteria and other impurities adhere to it. Tiny hair-like processes, or cilia,

■ **BOX 6.1 Colds**

If you have a cold, the lining of the nose becomes inflamed and secretes more mucus. You become aware of this mucus and call it catarrh. The infection can spread easily from the nose into the throat and sinuses of the skull because of the continuity of the mucous membrane lining the cavities.

project from the epithelium and have a lashing movement which moves the mucus in one direction, into the throat where it is swallowed. In this way the lining of the nose acts as a filter for the air.

The pharynx

The pharynx is the throat. It is a muscular tube about 12 cm long lying in front of the cervical vertebrae and behind the nose, the mouth and the larynx. It is lined with mucous membrane and is described in three parts: the nasopharynx, the oropharynx and the laryngopharynx (Fig. 6.1).

The *nasopharynx* is continuous with the cavity of the nose. The *pharyngotympanic auditory tubes*, which carry air to the middle ear, have openings into the nasopharynx. These tubes are essential for hearing. This part of the pharynx contains some lymphoid tissue, called the pharyngeal tonsils. These may be overgrown in young children, causing obstruction of the passage for air. The enlarged masses of lymphoid tissue are also called *adenoids* and are the reason why some children breathe through the mouth.

The *oropharynx* is separated from the cavity of the mouth by two folds of mucous membrane (called the *fauces*), hanging down from the soft palate. Between these folds lie the oral tonsils. A muscular projection of the palate lies in the middle of the arch formed by these folds. This is the *uvula*.

The *laryngopharynx* is the part which opens into both the larynx and the oesophagus. This makes the oral and laryngeal parts of the pharynx a common passage for food and air.

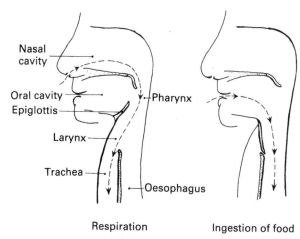

Nasal cavity
Oral cavity
Epiglottis
Larynx
Trachea
Pharynx
Oesophagus

Respiration   Ingestion of food

Fig. 6.2 Diagrammatic section of the pharynx.

If anything other than air enters the larynx, a cough reflex is initiated. This acts to expel the substance either through the mouth or into the oropharynx, where it can be safely swallowed. This protective reflex does not work when we are unconscious. If the obstruction is large and cannot be got rid of using the cough reflex, a manoeuvre called the Heimlich manoeuvre can be performed. This uses the air in the lungs of the choking person to expel the obstruction (usually a piece of food). All healthcare workers are advised to learn (by demonstration) this manoeuvre as it can be life saving.

If possible no food or drink is given approximately 4 hours prior to the administration of an anaesthetic. This is because the anaesthetic results in the loss of the cough and swallow reflexes. Some anaesthetics also irritate the stomach and can cause vomiting. If there is any food or fluid in the stomach it will pass into the pharynx and may enter the larynx and be inhaled into the lungs. This can result in death or, at the very least, initiate a chest infection.

Air passes from the nose down the nasopharynx, the oropharynx and the laryngopharynx into the larynx. Food passes from the mouth through the oropharynx and laryngopharynx into the oesophagus (Fig. 6.2). Once food, mucus and saliva have passed through the fauces into the pharynx, swallowing becomes an involuntary action. If breathing takes place while food is in the pharynx, it will be inhaled into the larynx and cause choking, which we describe as 'food going down the wrong way.' To prevent this happening, the entrance to the nasopharynx constricts and prevents the food from going up into the nose. The *epiglottis* (part of the larynx) closes the inlet to the larynx and food is directed down into the oesophagus.

The larynx

As well as being an air passage, the larynx is the voice box. It can be felt at the top of the neck and is made of several cartilages joined by ligaments. The largest of these cartilages is the *thyroid* cartilage. It consists of two plates of hyaline cartilage fused together in front but incomplete at the back, rather like a partly opened book. Below the thyroid cartilage is the *cricoid* cartilage which is shaped like a signet ring. The wide part of the ring lies posteriorly and fits in between the plates of the thyroid cartilage. Situated at the top of the posterior part of the cricoid are two small *arytenoid* cartilages. These cartilages have the vocal cords attached to them. The fourth cartilage is the *epiglottis*. It is a leaf-shaped structure attached to the inner surface of the thyroid cartilage. During swallowing, the larynx rises and the epiglottis covers over the inlet (see Figs 6.1 and 6.2).

The voice

The larynx is lined with mucous membrane which becomes ciliated in the lower part. In the upper part, two folds of this membrane form the *vocal cords*. These cords stretch across from the thyroid cartilage in front to the arytenoid cartilages at the back, narrowing the air passage. As air from the lungs is forced through the cords the voice is produced. The brain, the tongue, the lips, the facial muscles and the air sinuses all help to convert these sounds into speech.

The vocal cords can be tightened or slackened like a violin string to give pitch to the voice. At puberty a boy's larynx will enlarge with the result that the vocal cords are longer than a girl's. His voice is said to 'break', producing a lower pitch. This larger larynx in a man is sometimes very prominent and is called his 'Adam's apple'.

The loudness of the voice depends on the amount of air which is forced through the cords making them vibrate. The resonance and quality of the voice depend on the hollow air sinuses in the skull, the shape of the mouth and the position of the tongue.

■ **BOX 6.2 Laryngitis**

Laryngitis is inflammation of the larynx. The vocal cords become swollen and the voice becomes a whisper. In sinusitis the voice loses its resonance.

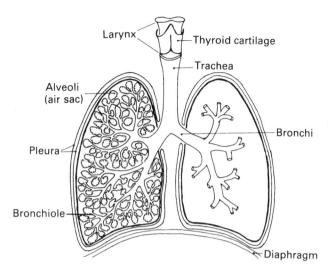

Fig. 6.3 Air passages and lungs.

Essential oils are volatile substances – when they evaporate their vapours may be inhaled. Therefore, they have direct access to the respiratory system.

Many of the essential oils used in aromatherapy can aid the respiratory system, e.g. *expectorant* and *mucolytic* oils are used in cases of congestion, *balsamic* and *antitussive* oils are useful for coughs and irritation, while many oils act as respiratory *antiseptics* and can help combat infection.

The trachea

The trachea is the windpipe. It is continuous with the larynx and is about 10 cm long. It consists of C-shaped cartilages joined by muscle and fibrous tissue. The rings of cartilage can be felt in front of the neck. The back of the trachea is soft and lies anterior to the oesophagus. It is lined with ciliated mucous membrane.

The bronchi

At about the middle of the thorax the trachea divides to form the right and left bronchus. The bronchi enter the lungs, the right one dividing into three and the left one into two branches (Fig. 6.3).

Irritants which have been inhaled may cause an excess of mucus to be secreted. When it is coughed up, this mucus may be thin and watery or thick and sticky. We call it *sputum* and the act of coughing it up is called expectoration.

These branches divide again and again getting smaller each time. The bronchi have a similar structure to the trachea except that the rings of cartilage are complete.

If you study Figure 6.3 you will see that the system of air passages looks like an inverted tree. The trachea is the trunk and the bronchi the limbs and branches. The twigs of the bronchial tree are the *bronchioles* which are the smallest of the air passages. The bronchioles lie entirely within the lungs and have no cartilagenous rings. They consist of involuntary muscle tissue and elastic fibrous tissue. From the trachea right down to the smallest bronchiole the lining is ciliated mucous membrane.

The bronchioles end in *alveolar* ducts and *alveoli* (Fig. 6.4). These are thin-walled air sacs consisting of squamous epithelium. They are like balloons and are surrounded by a network of capillaries from the pulmonary circulation. This is where the interchange of gases takes place.

The air is moistened and warmed as it passes down the bronchial tree. The cilia moves the mucus, with any inhaled particles, up out of the lungs into the pharynx where it is swallowed.

The rings of cartilage in the bronchi hold the passages open. The muscular walls of the bronchioles, however, are under nervous control. When they contract the passage becomes narrow and when they relax the passage is dilated.

■ BOX 6.3 Asthma, chronic bronchitis, emphysema

In allergic conditions such as *asthma*, the muscular wall goes into spasm, the mucous lining becomes oedematous, the patient has difficulty in breathing and becomes very distressed. Chronic *bronchitis* and *emphysema* are other common diseases which obstruct the airway. The mucous lining is inflamed and swollen, obstructing the air flow, and the alveoli become distended with air which is trapped in them.

THE LUNGS

The lungs are cone-shaped spongy organs situated in the thorax on either side of the heart. As the heart lies slightly over towards the left side, the left lung is smaller than the right one. The base of each lung rests on the diaphragm and the apex extends up into the neck just behind the clavicle.

Each lung consists of lobes and each lobe is made up of lobules. There are three lobes in the right lung and two lobes in the left lung. On the medial side of each lung there is a depression called the hilus. This is where the bronchus, pulmonary artery, bronchial artery and nerves enter the lung and the two pulmonary veins, the bronchial veins and the lymphatic vessels leave. Each lung is made up of all these structures along with the branches of the bronchi, the bronchioles and the alveoli. Elastic connective tissue forms a delicate network holding the various parts together.

The pleura

On the outside of each lung is a serous membrane called the pleura. This membrane is a double sac. The outer (parietal) layer lines the chest wall and covers the upper surface of the diaphragm. The inner (visceral) layer is attached to the surface of the lung and these two layers are always in con-

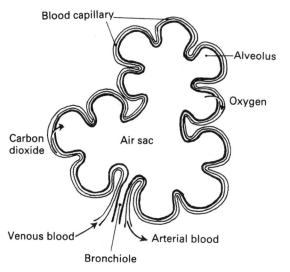

Fig. 6.4 An air sac.

■ **BOX 6.4 Pleurisy**

Inflammation of the pleura is called *pleurisy*. In pleurisy pain is experienced at the end of a deep inspiration when the pleura is stretched and there is friction between the inflamed surfaces.

tact. The pleura secretes a serous fluid which lies between the two layers and prevents them from rubbing on each other during breathing. The pleura can slide across one another but their separation is strongly resisted by the surface tension of the pleural fluid between them. Therefore, the lungs cling tightly to the chest wall and are forced to expand and recoil passively as the size of the chest cavity increases and decreases with inspiration and expiration.

THE MECHANISM OF BREATHING

Breathing is the passage of air in and out of the lungs. This occurs about 12 to 16 times each minute. The amount of air going in and out is called the *tidal volume* and is about 400 ml. During the deepest possible inspiration the amount of air taken in is about 4000 ml and is called the *vital capacity*.

The muscles responsible for breathing are the *diaphragm* and the *intercostal* muscles. The diaphragm forms the dome-shaped floor of the thorax. It flattens out when it contracts, thus increasing the depth of the thorax on inspiration. At the same time the intercostal muscles contract and raise the ribs upwards and outwards. The thorax is increased in size in all directions and air passes in through the air passages (Fig. 6.5). The lungs stretch because of their elasticity and fill up the space created. On expiration, the diaphragm and intercostal muscles relax, pressure is exerted on the elastic

Breathing can become impaired by stress and anxiety, so any of the therapies that help reduce stress and induce relaxation will be beneficial. Relaxation programmes, including meditation techniques, focus on breathing patterns as a means to alter the state of mind, inducing calmness and also physical relaxation.

Massage can increase the vital capacity of the lungs by reducing tightness of the muscles and fascia that are involved in breathing. Some massage manipulations such as *tapotement* (percussion) and *vibration* can be used to help loosen and discharge phlegm in the respiratory tract.

Patients who have undergone abdominal surgery may not cough adequately because it hurts the wound, and so they risk developing postoperative pneumonia. In this condition, inflammation of the alveoli occurs as a result of failure to clear the mucus from the lungs.

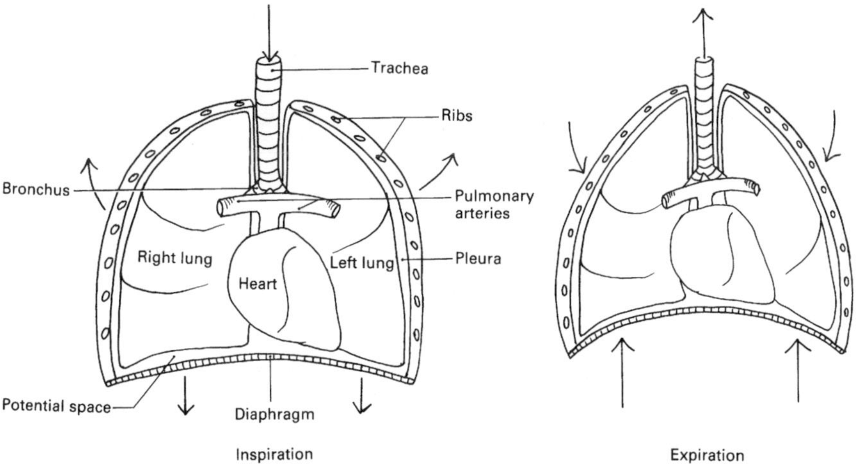

Fig. 6.5 Diagrammatic representation of the mechanism of breathing. Diaphragm and lungs.

Patients suffering from dyspnoea (difficulty in breathing) should be nursed in the upright position and may be given a bed table to lean on. This allows for fixation of the shoulder girdle and use of the shoulder muscles to help raise the chest. This makes breathing a little easier.

The respirations are one of the commonly recorded observations carried out by healthcare workers. The rate, depth and pattern of a client's respiration are all noted over the period of one full minute. Normal breathing is effortless, automatic, regular and quiet. Any deviations from normal should be investigated.

lungs, they recoil and air is expelled. There is always about 1500 ml of air left in the lungs at the end of expiration. This is called the *residual volume*.

Other muscles are involved in deep or difficult breathing. These are the abdominal muscles and some of the neck and shoulder girdle muscles.

Control of breathing is rather complex and is mainly under the control of the brain. We can alter our breathing, during singing or speaking, for example, but only for a short time before involuntary control takes over. If breathing stops for more than 3 minutes, permanent brain damage or even death will result. However, if you try holding your breath you will find that long before the 3 minutes are up an involuntary expiration has taken place.

There are special respiratory centres formed of nerve cells which control the rate and depth of our breaths. These are found in the brainstem, in particular, the medulla oblongata and the pons varolii. Motor impulses leaving these centres pass through the phrenic and intercostal nerves to innervate the muscles of respiration, the diaphragm and the intercostal muscles.

There are also receptors, in particular chemoreceptors, which monitor changes in oxygen and carbon dioxide levels in the blood. These are located centrally in the brain and peripherally in the arch of the aorta and the carotid arteries. These receptors stimulate the respiratory centre via nerves, and the rate and depth of breathing is increased or decreased in order to bring blood gas levels back to normal. Rising carbon dioxide levels are the most powerful respiratory stimulant and the level of arterial carbon dioxide is maintained between very narrow limits. Increased muscle action produces more carbon dioxide, therefore exercise will increase the rate and depth of respiration.

■ BOX 6.5 Hypoxia

Hypoxia is a lack of oxygen being delivered to the tissues of the body and may have many causes. It can be easily seen in fair-skinned people as their skin and mucosa take on a bluish tint (cyanosis). However, in people with a darker skin tone this change in colour may only be seen in the mucosa and the nail beds.

RESPIRATORY SYSTEM QUESTIONS

Diagrams—Questions 266–278

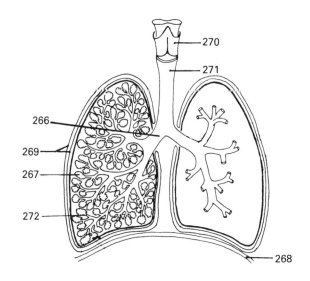

266–272. The air passages and lungs

A. Trachea
B. Right bronchus
C. Bronchioles
D. Alveoli
E. Pleura
F. Thyroid cartilage
G. Diaphragm

| 266 |
| 267 |
| 268 |
| 269 |
| 270 |
| 271 |
| 272 |

273–278. Section through head and neck

A. Uvula
B. Pharynx
C. Epiglottis
D. Oesophagus
E. Larynx
F. Hyoid bone

| 273 |
| 274 |
| 275 |
| 276 |
| 277 |
| 278 |

Questions 279–286 are of the multiple choice type

279. The amount of air entering and leaving the lungs during normal respiration is: 279
A. 200 ml
B. 400 ml
C. 2000 ml
D. 4000 ml.

280. The percentage of oxygen in inspired air is: 280
A. 16%
B. 20%
C. 0.04%
D. 78%.

281. The percentage of nitrogen in expired air is: 281
A. 16%
B. 20%
C. 60%
D. 78%.

282. The conchae are: 282
A. part of the lung
B. part of the larynx
C. bones in the nose
D. the openings into the sinuses.

283. The pharyngotympanic tubes open into one of the following: 283
A. the nose
B. the nasopharynx
C. the oropharynx
D. the laryngopharynx.

284. The lining of the nasal sinuses is: 284
A. cuboid epithelium
B. ciliated epithelium
C. squamous epithelium
D. transitional epithelium.

285. Resonance of the voice depends on the: 285
A. force of air from the lungs
B. tension in the vocal chords
C. nasal sinuses
D. position of the uvula.

286. The left bronchus: 286
A. lies just above the diaphragm
B. recoils during expiration
C. has C-shaped rings of cartilage
D. divides into two branches.

Questions 287–318 are of the true/false type   T | F

287–290. The adenoids are:
   287. laryngeal cartilages
   288. lymphoid tissue
   289. oral tonsils
   290. pharyngeal tonsils.

291–294. The vocal cords are attached to the:
   291. thyroid cartilage
   292. cricoid cartilage
   293. arytenoid cartilage
   294. epiglottis.

295–298. The trachea:
   295. is lined with ciliated mucous membrane
   296. is made of involuntary muscle tissue only
   297. joins the larynx to the bronchioles
   298. lies in front of the oesophagus.

299–302. The bronchioles are:
   299. made of cartilage
   300. made of muscle tissue
   301. lined with squamous epithelium
   302. lined with ciliated columnar epithelium.

303–306. The lungs:
   303. are identical in size
   304. have no lymphatic vessels
   305. lie in one pleural cavity
   306. contain a great deal of elastic tissue.

307–310. In the lungs:
   307. mucus is moved upwards by peristalsis
   308. expiration is the result of recoil of the elastic tissue
   309. the parietal layer of the pleura remains in contact with the visceral layer
   310. the pulmonary artery contains oxygenated blood.

311–314. The alveoli:
   311. are made of squamous epithelium
   312. are lined with ciliated columnar epithelium
   313. are surrounded by capillaries from the bronchial artery
   314. recoil during expiration.

315–318. The diaphragm:
   315. has several openings in it
   316. is dome-shaped during inspiration
   317. flattens when it contracts
   318. forms the roof of the abdomen.

Questions 319–324 are of the matching items type

319–321. From the list on the left select a sign or symptom of each disease on the right.

A. the walls of the bronchi constrict	319. asthma	319
B. the alveoli are distended	320. emphysema	320
C. expiration is difficult and painful	321. pleurisy.	321
D. there is pain on inspiration		
E. the walls of the bronchioles go into spasm		

322–324. From the list on the left select the volume of air involved in the list on the right.

A. 250 ml	322. residual air	322
B. 400 ml	323. tidal air	323
C. 1500 ml	324. vital capacity.	324
D. 4000 ml		
E. 4500 ml		

The digestive system

7

■ KEY POINTS

- Food and its uses
- Structure and function of the digestive tract
- The mouth
- The pharynx
- The oesophagus
- The stomach
- The small intestine
- Peritoneum
- The large intestine
- The liver
- The biliary system
- The pancreas
- Metabolism.

INTRODUCTION

The digestive system consists of all the organs that are concerned in the breakdown, digestion and absorption of nutrients and the elimination of the residue.

It consists of the digestive tract and the accessory organs of digestion (see Fig. 7.1).

CONSTITUENTS OF FOOD

The body needs food to provide energy. Vitamins and minerals are necessary to maintain good health. The main food groups are carbohydrate, fat and protein. In addition, water is essential to replace fluid which is continually being lost, and roughage is required for optimal absorption and to aid elimination. There are, in total, six essential foodstuffs with which the body must be constantly supplied (Box 7.1), each of which will be examined in turn.

These foodstuffs must be digested and absorbed. Food must therefore be of such a nature that it can be digested, i.e. broken down by digestive juices into substances that can pass into the bloodstream and be carried to various tissues for their use.

■ BOX 7.1 Essential foodstuffs

- Protein
- Carbohydrate
- Fat
- Water
- Mineral salts
- Vitamins.

Carbohydrates

The food required for energy and heat within the body is called carbohydrate because it contains carbon, hydrogen and oxygen. Carbohydrates include sugar and starch and they are the chief source of body fuel.

Fats

Fatty foods also provide energy and heat which serve as body fuel. They also provide food stores – the adipose tissue of the body and protective coverings for some organs.

Proteins

Proteins are the most complicated of the foodstuffs. Protein foods contain nitrogen in addition to hydrogen, carbon, oxygen and, in some cases, sulphur and phosphorus. They are called nitrogenous foodstuffs, as they are the only ones that contain the element nitrogen. Protein is necessary in the diet to build and replace the protoplasm of body cells. Proteins are composed of polypeptides, which are long chains of amino acids. There are 20 amino acids, although each protein contains only some of these. Humans require approximately 0.75 g of protein per kg of body weight per day.

Water

Signs of dehydration:
- thirst
- dry mouth
- slack, inelastic skin
- sunken eyes
- low blood pressure.

Water is absolutely essential for life as it forms nearly two-thirds of the human body and is present in most of the foods we eat. The average amount of water in the human body is about 45 litres (30 litres inside the cells – intracellular – and 15 litres outside the cells as extracellular fluid). The purpose of water in the body is summarized in Box. 7.2. If the body is depleted of fluid, the signs and symptoms of dehydration may appear.

The body requires 2–3 litres of water every day and the amount of fluid taken into the body must be balanced by the output.

Mineral salts

Minerals are salts which are essential for normal metabolism. Salts are produced by the action of an acid on a mineral.

An electrolyte is a dissolved salt (a mineral salt) which is capable of conducting electricity. The two major electrolytes in the body are sodium (Na^+) and potassium (K^+). The concentration of Na^+ is high in extracellular sites and low within cells (intracellular). In contrast K^+ ions are low in tissue fluids and high within cells. A correct balance of electrolytes is essential for normal function of body tissues and fluids.

■ BOX 7.2 Purpose of water in the body

- Excretion of waste products
- Making of digestive and lubricating fluids
- Building of body tissues and body fluids
- Temperature control (i.e. evaporation of sweat).

■ **BOX 7.3 Ions and electrolytes**

Ion = charged particle, e.g. Na^+, Cl^-.

Electrolyte = an ionic compound in solution in water; can conduct electricity, e.g. sodium chloride.

Sodium is present in all tissues; it exists as sodium chloride at a concentration of 9 grams per litre (0.9%) in all extracellular fluids. Sodium is derived from our food, particularly animal foodstuffs, from salt used in cooking and in processed foods.

Potassium is present in all tissue cells. It is obtained from food, particularly plant foodstuffs.

Calcium is present in all tissues, particularly in bone, in teeth and in blood, and it is necessary for the functioning of nerves and muscles. It is obtained chiefly from milk, cheese, eggs and green vegetables.

Iron is essential for the formation of the haemoglobin in red blood cells. It is obtained from green vegetables, particularly spinach and cabbage, egg yolk and red meats. Men require 10 mg daily; women require more (10–15 mg daily) because of menstrual blood loss.

Iodine is required for the formation of thyroxine by the thyroid gland. It is obtained from seafood and is also present in green vegetables.

Vitamins

Vitamins are substances which are also essential to normal health, because they are necessary for a range of metabolic functions; they are of no value to the body as a fuel or as building material. Vitamins are present in small quantities in foodstuffs and are only required in minute traces each day. Vitamins are classified as fat soluble and water soluble; vitamins A, D, E and K are fat soluble, the other vitamins, including B and C, are soluble in water.

Vitamin A is present in all fatty foods, i.e. milk, cheese and fish liver oils. It can be made in the body from a substance called carotene which is present in carrots and tomatoes. Vitamin A is needed for normal function of the retina and to fight infection. Correspondingly, a lack of vitamin A causes visual loss, stunted growth and a lowered resistance to infection.

Vitamin D is found in dairy produce and also in fatty fish, such as herring. Cod liver oil and halibut liver oil are very rich in vitamin D. Vitamin D can also be built up in the body, the ultraviolet rays from the sun act on a fatty substance in the skin which produces vitamin D. Vitamin D is necessary, with calcium, for the formation of bone. Lack of vitamin D and/ or calcium leads to rickets in childhood, osteomalacia and osteoporosis in adults.

Vitamin E is present in vegetable oils and is found in egg yolk and milk. It is necessary for normal functions of the nervous system, reproduction and muscle development, and acts as an antioxidant, preventing damage to tissues caused by reactive oxidizing agents.

Vitamin K is fat soluble and can be obtained from green vegetables and liver. It is required for the production of blood clotting factors in the liver. Vitamin K is also synthesized in the intestine by colonic bacterial action.

■ BOX 7.4 Scurvy

Lack of vitamin C causes scurvy, a condition which used to be common in sailors on long sea voyages. Scurvy is occasionally seen today in elderly people who have not been feeding themselves properly.

Vitamin B is a complex of several closely related compounds. These are found particularly in the husks and germs of cereals and pulses, in yeast and yeast extracts and to a lesser extent in vegetables, fruit, milk, eggs and meat. The chief factors in the vitamin B complex are:

- *vitamin B_1* (thiamine), essential for carbohydrate metabolism and controls the nutrition of nerve cells
- *vitamin B_2* (riboflavin) is essential for the proper functioning of cell enzymes
- *vitamin B_6* (pyridoxine) is necessary for protein metabolism
- *vitamin B_{12}* (cyanocobalamin) is the anti-anaemic substance or factor absorbed by the villi of the small intestine and stored in the liver; it is satisfactorily absorbed only in the presence of intrinsic factor produced by the cells in the lining of the stomach. Vitamin B_{12} is essential for the proper development of red cells in the red bone marrow and of nervous tissue
- *folic acid* is required in the body for the maturation of red blood cells; it is derived from green vegetables.

Vitamin C (ascorbic acid) is water soluble and is found in citrus fruits (oranges, grapefruits and lemons), green vegetables and potatoes. Vitamin C is important in tissue respiratory activity, wound repair and resistance to infection, and it affects the condition of capillary walls. It is also an antioxidant (see Vitamin E).

Roughage

Roughage is an indigestible part of food, it remains in the bowel and stimulates it to empty itself. Roughage is the fibrous part of food, giving it bulk and stimulating bowel action, thus preventing constipation.

STRUCTURE AND FUNCTION OF THE DIGESTIVE TRACT

The gastrointestinal (GI) tract takes in, breaks down and absorbs food and fluids. It consists of a digestive tract, a tube extending from mouth to the anus, and its associated accessory organs, primarily glands, which secrete fluids into the digestive tract (Fig. 7.1).

At various points of the GI tract, food is mixed with digestive juices. These juices contain digestive *enzymes*. These enzymes are chemical substances which break down complex proteins, carbohydrates and fats into substances which are easier to digest and absorb.

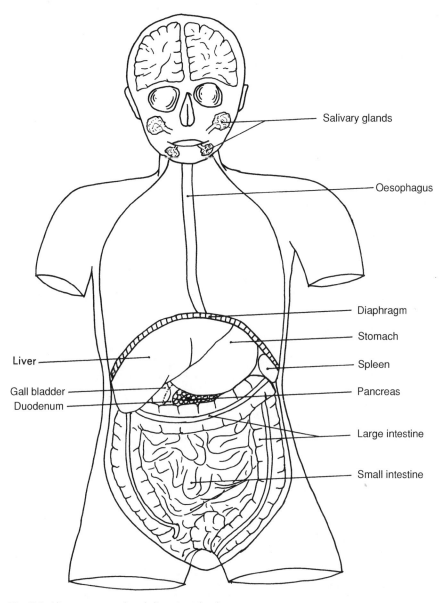

Fig. 7.1 Alimentary canal and digestive glands.

■ **BOX 7.5 The digestive tract**

- Oesophagus
- Stomach
- Small intestine
- Large intestine.

■ **BOX 7.6 Accessory organs of the GI tract**

- Salivary glands
- Liver and bile ducts
- Gall bladder
- Pancreas.

Structure of the gastrointestinal tract: an overview

The digestive tract wall consists of four structural layers (Box 7.7, Fig. 7.2). These four layers are present in all areas of the tract from the oesophagus to the anus, with some functional adaptations throughout.

The *mucosa* is the innermost layer, that is, the layer nearest to the lumen of the tube, and it exhibits a great deal of variation throughout the tract. Stratified epithelial cells line the lumen (except oesophagus), and it is from this layer that all glands develop. Mucus-secreting cells are situated throughout the epithelium. These cells are subjected to a tremendous

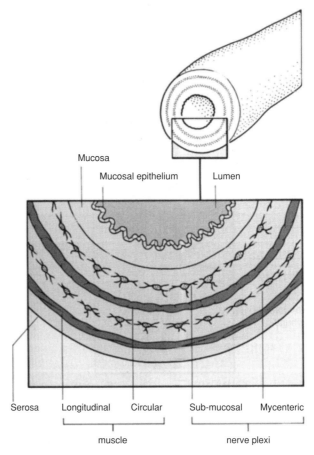

Fig. 7.2 Basic structure of the digestive tract (from Rutishauser S. Physiology and anatomy: a basis for nursing and health care. Edinburgh: Churchill Livingstone; 1994).

■ BOX 7.7 Generalized layers of the gasrointestinal tract

- Mucosa
- Submucosa
- Muscularis
- Serosa (fibrous outer layer).

amount of frictional wear and tear. The epithelial cells lie on a sheet of connective tissue called the *lamina propria*. Distal to this, there is a thin layer of muscle tissue called *muscularis mucosa*. Throughout the mucosa are patches of lymphoid tissue which serve a defensive function.

The *submucosa* lies distal to the mucosa, and consists of loose connective tissue which supports blood vessels, lymphatics and nerve fibres. The *muscularis* layer, as its name suggests, is formed of smooth muscle fibres. The *serosa* is the outermost, protective layer, formed of connective tissue and squamous serous epithelium, containing many elastic fibres.

THE MOUTH

The mouth can be divided into two parts:

1. The *vestibule:* the part between the teeth and the jaws, and the lips and cheeks. The salivary glands open here.
2. The *oral cavity:* the inner area which is bounded by the teeth. The epithelium in the oral cavity is typically 15–20 layers of cells thick, and as such is adapted to the amount of friction that occurs during mastication (Fig. 7.3).

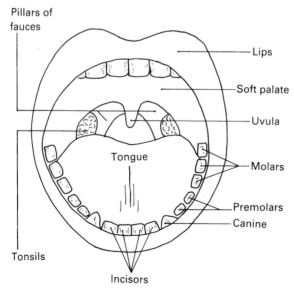

Fig. 7.3 The mouth.

The teeth

The teeth break down food mechanically. The *incisors* and *canines* are sharp teeth in the front. These teeth bite, cut and tear up the food into little pieces. At the back of the mouth are the larger, flat teeth, the *premolars* and the *molars*. The teeth are embedded in sockets in the gum. There are 32 permanent teeth and 20 temporary ones. Permanent teeth start to replace the temporary ones from about the age of 6 years, in a process usually completed by the twenty-fifth year. Each tooth has two parts; the crown, which is above the gum, and the root, which is in the tooth socket. The incisors and canines have one root but others can have two or three roots (Fig. 7.4).

Teeth are made of *dentine*, a hard yellowish-white tissue. The outer layer is in two parts; that covering the crown is the *enamel* and is a hard, white layer, while that covering the root is called *cement* and is a thin layer, resembling bone in structure. The root is fixed in the socket by cement. In the centre of each tooth is a cavity, the pulp cavity, which contains blood vessels and nerves. From infancy onwards, it is important that our diet contains sufficient calcium, phosphorus and vitamins C and D to keep teeth healthy.

The tongue

The tongue is a muscular organ lying on the floor of the mouth, it is attached to the mandible and to a small bone called the hyoid bone. In certain areas of the tongue the mucous membrane is modified, forming projections (called *papillae*) which increase the surface area. These projections contain microscopic taste buds, which are widespread over almost the entire area of the tongue. The taste buds are the endings of the nerves of

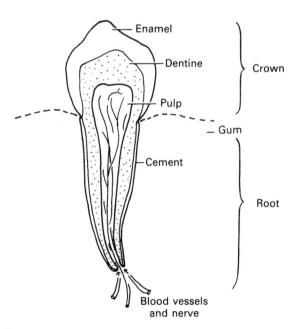

Fig. 7.4 A tooth.

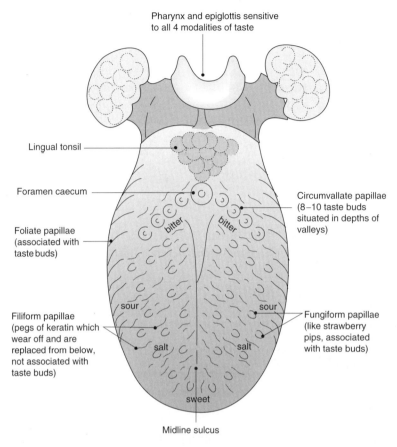

Pharynx and epiglottis sensitive
to all 4 modalities of taste

Lingual tonsil

Foramen caecum

Circumvallate papillae
(8–10 taste buds
situated in depths of
valleys)

Foliate papillae
(associated with
taste buds)

bitter   bitter

sour   sour

Filiform papillae
(pegs of keratin which
wear off and are
replaced from below,
not associated with
taste buds)

salt   salt

Fungiform papillae
(like strawberry
pips, associated
with taste buds)

sweet

Midline sulcus

Fig. 7.5 The tongue and taste buds (from Cheshire E. Crash course: gastrointestinal system. London: Mosby–Wolfe; 1997).

taste and give the sensations of salt, sweet, sour or bitter of any substance that can be dissolved in water (Fig. 7.5). The main functions of the tongue are:

- taste
- mastication of food
- swallowing
- speech.

The salivary glands

There are three main pairs of salivary glands situated around the mouth (Fig. 7.6). There are numerous smaller glands scattered throughout the mouth. The *parotid* gland is the largest and lies just below the ear; its duct is about 5 cm long and enters into the mouth on the inside of the cheek. The *submandibular* and *sublingual* glands both open into the floor of the mouth. The salivary glands are supplied by the autonomic nervous system (ANS) and the secretion of saliva is stimulated by the sight, smell or thought of food, a conditioned (or learned) reflex.

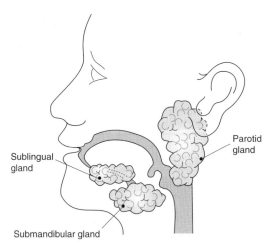

Fig. 7.6 The main paired salivary glands (from Cheshire E. Crash course: gastrointestinal system. London: Mosby–Wolfe; 1997).

> Dysphagia is defined as difficulty in swallowing. Patients may be able to swallow soft foods and liquids but may be unable to take more solid foodstuffs. Dysphagia may be due to mechanical obstruction (i.e. oesophageal cancer), dysfunction in the neuromuscular structures involved in swallowing or to diseases of the mouth, larynx and pharynx.

Saliva

Water makes up 90–95% of saliva, the remaining 5–10% being dissolved solutes. These include:

- ions (bicarbonate, chloride, phosphate, sodium and potassium)
- the enzyme salivary amylase
- lysozymes
- organic substances (urea, albumins and globulins)
- mucin derived from mucus-secreting cells.

THE PHARYNX

The pharynx is a muscular tube approximately 14 cm in length. Once food has been chewed and moistened the tongue rolls it into a *bolus* and carries it towards the oral part of the pharynx. When the bolus reaches the pharynx, swallowing begins. The muscular wall of the pharynx constricts and pushes the food over the epiglottis (which closes the larynx), and on into the oesophagus.

THE OESOPHAGUS

The oesophagus is a muscular canal about 25 cm long extending from the pharynx to the stomach. The layers of the oesophagus are essentially the same as the other parts of the GI tract (see Box 7.7). The mucosal lining of the normal oesophagus is mainly stratified squamous epithelium. The muscular coat of the upper two-thirds of the oesophagus is of striped voluntary muscle; the lower one-third contains smooth muscle. The oesophagus is innervated by the vagus (Xth cranial) nerve. Movement of food through the oesophagus is by peristaltic action. Peristalsis occurs as a

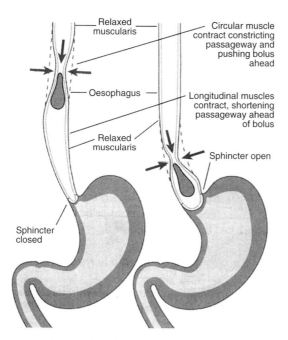

Fig. 7.7 The movement of materials in the oesophagus (from Hinchcliff SM, Montague SE, Watson R. Physiology for nursing practice. London: Ballière Tindall; 1996).

The symptoms of heartburn and acid indigestion are caused by a backflow of acidic stomach contents into the oesophagus causing sensations of burning and pressure behind the breastbone. In its simplest form gastro-oesophageal reflux disease (GORD) symptoms are mild and occur infrequently and may respond to simple non-pharmaceutical interventions including avoiding problem foods, stopping smoking, reducing alcohol intake or losing weight. In more severe cases, acid-blocking medications (H_2 receptor antagonists) or more powerful inhibitors of stomach acid production (proton pump inhibitors) may be required to treat the symptoms.

response to stretching of the smooth muscle layer of the tract, it involves contraction of circular muscles, followed by a contraction of the adjacent distal longitudinal fibres while the circular fibres relax. These movements occur progressively throughout the tube in a coordinated manner, to produce a smooth wave of contraction.

An upper oesophageal sphincter and lower (cardiac) sphincter, at the upper and lower ends of the oesophagus, respectively, regulate the movement of materials into and out of the oesophagus (Fig. 7.7).

THE STOMACH

The stomach, continuous with the oesophagus above and the duodenum below, is the most dilated area of the GI tract. It is a muscular organ which is roughly J-shaped, although size and shape may vary between individuals and with its state of fullness. The capacity of the stomach is about 1500 ml in the adult. Its internal surface area has visible folds, called *rugae*, which, together with the muscle layer, allows distension of the stomach. The muscular layer of the stomach varies from other regions of the GI tract in that it consists of three layers of smooth muscle fibres, the outer being longitudinal, the middle being circular and the inner being oblique. The upper opening of the stomach is called the *cardiac orifice* and the lower opening, into the duodenum, is called the *pylorus*, guarded by the *pyloric sphincter* which prevents the regurgitation of food from the duodenum into the stomach.

■ **BOX 7.8 Hiatal hernia**

A hiatal hernia is a widening of the oesophageal opening, occurring most commonly in adults, which allows part of the stomach to extend through the opening into the thorax. This allows gastro-oesophageal reflux to occur causing irritation and possibly narrowing of the oesophagus in the longer term.

Figure 7.8 illustrates the four main regions of the stomach, which are:

1. The cardiac (cardia) region; surrounds the cardiac sphincter muscle.
2. The fundic (fundus) region; the elevated rounded portion, to the left of the cardiac portion.
3. The body region; occupies most of the stomach and lies between the fundic and pyloric regions.
4. The pyloric (pylorus) region: the inferior part of the stomach, lying superior to the pyloric sphincter.

The main functions of the stomach are:

- mechanical breakdown of food (churn)
- chemical digestion of food by means of the gastric juice
- secretion of intrinsic factor.

The stomach's secretion is called gastric juice, which is produced from gastric glands in the gastric pits. Each gastric gland possesses three main types of specialized secretory cells, which secrete the separate components of gastric juice. These cells are:

1. *Mucous cells*. These secrete mucus which protects the mucous membrane from the action of gastric juice.

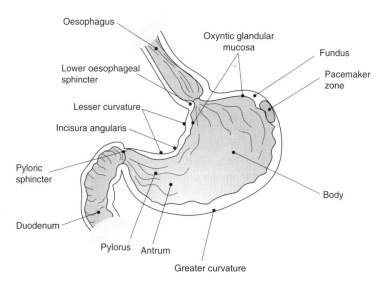

Fig. 7.8 The stomach (from Cheshire E. Crash course: gastrointestinal system. London: Mosby–Wolfe; 1997).

■ BOX 7.9 Contents of gastric juice

- Water and mineral salts
- Mucus
- Hydrochloric acid (HCl)
- Pepsinogen (inactive precursor to the enzyme pepsin)
- Prorennin (inactive precursor to the enzyme rennin).

2. *Chief (zymogen) cells* secrete two enzyme precursors (inactive enzymes) which are activated by the acidic gastric juice to pepsin and renin. Pepsin acts in the presence of hydrochloric acid to break down protein molecules into polypeptides.
3. *Parietal (oxyntic) cells* secrete hydrochloric acid. This acid aids digestion and kills potentially harmful bacteria which may have been swallowed with food. Intrinsic factor, which is essential for the absorption of vitamin B_{12}, is also produced by parietal cells.

The secretion of gastric juice occurs in response to the presence or anticipation of food. Three phases are responsible for controlling the secretion of gastric juice. They are referred to as the *cephalic phase*, the *gastric phase* and the *intestinal phase*. The gastric glands are also stimulated by an internal secretion or hormone, produced by the stomach, called *gastrin*, which passes into the circulation, and when it reaches the gastric glands increases the production of gastric juice.

Acid secretion is mediated by three mechanisms:

- the autonomic nervous system via the vagus nerve
- the chemical histamine produced by mast cells in the stomach
- the production of gastrin, a hormone produced by 'G' cells in the stomach in response to an increased gastric pH.

The most important function of the stomach is to act as a reservoir for ingested food and to then regulate the passage of its contents into the duodenum. Peristaltic activity within the stomach churns the contents, and when the ingested food particles are reduced to a critical size the pylorus permits their passage into the duodenum. The churning action of the stomach converts foodstuff into a greyish-white fluid called *chyme*. Food will normally remain in the stomach for $\frac{1}{2}$ hour to 3 hours or more, according to the nature of the food and the muscularity of the individual stomach.

THE SMALL INTESTINE

The small intestine consists of a long coiled tube; its structure closely follows the generalized structure of the GI tract (see Fig. 7.2). The small intestine extends from the pyloric sphincter to its junction with the large intestine at the ileo-caecal valve (Fig. 7.9). The small intestine is about 5 metres long in a living person and most of it is attached to the posterior

Irritable bowel syndrome (IBS) is a functional bowel disorder in which abdominal pain is associated with defaecation or a change in bowel habit. Typically the bowel habit is chaotic – sometimes constipation, sometimes diarrhoea, sometimes both in the same day. The aetiology of IBS is unknown, although it is postulated that it is closely related to stress and therefore stress management programmes and supportive psychological therapies, such as hypnotherapy, may well reduce the stress response and lead to symptomatic improvements.

Vomiting results in the rapid expulsion of the stomach contents through the mouth. It is initiated and coordinated by the nervous system. When the descent of the diaphragm coincides with the contraction of the abdominal muscles, the rise in abdominal pressure forces the gastric contents out through the mouth. Integration of the vomiting sequence occurs in a vomiting centre in the brainstem.

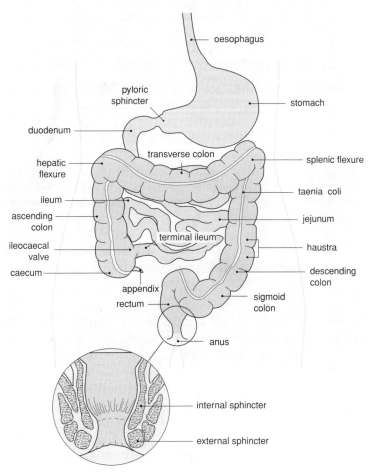

Fig. 7.9 The position of the small and large intestines (from Cheshire E. Crash course: gastrointestinal system. London: Mosby–Wolfe; 1997).

abdominal wall by a double fold of serous membrane called *peritoneum*. The small intestine consists of the duodenum, jejunum and ileum.

The mucosal surface of the small intestine is covered with many finger-like processes called *villi* (singular; villus), each of which contains a central lymph channel, called a *lacteal*, and a network of capillaries. Each villus is covered with a single layer of specialized epithelial cells. The villi contain two main cell types: the *goblet cells*, secreting mucus, and the *enterocytes*, which are involved in both digestion and absorption. The surface area is further increased with the presence of *microvilli* (microscopic finger-like processes). The *duodenum* is a short (25 cm long), C-shaped portion which lies mostly behind the peritoneum. Ducts from the gall bladder and liver and the pancreas enter directly into the duodenum via the *hepato-pancreatic ampulla (ampulla of Vater)*, which is guarded by a sphincter like muscle, the hepato-pancreatic sphincter (*sphincter of Oddi*) (see Fig. 7.12). When food from the stomach enters the duodenum, hormones are released which

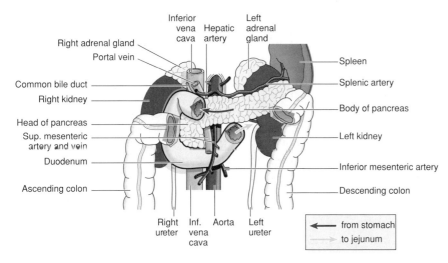

Fig. 7.10 The duodenum and associated structures (after Waugh A, Grant A. Ross and Wilson Anatomy and physiology in health and illness. 9th edn. Edinburgh: Churchill Livingstone; 2001).

simultaneously stimulate the release of bile from the gall bladder and pancreatic juice from the pancreas. In addition, the entry of food into the duodenum also stimulates the nervous *enterogastric reflex*, which has an inhibitory effect on the stomach.

The *jejunum* is the name given to the upper two-fifths of the remainder of the small intestine, and the lower three-fifths is called the *ileum*. Intestinal juice is secreted by the jejunum and ileum, the enzymes in intestinal juice are mostly contained in the enterocytes of the walls of the villi and are responsible for the completion of digestion. Three litres of intestinal juice, with a pH of 7.8–8.0, are normally produced each day by the small intestine in response to local mechanical stimuli and the chemical stimuli of partially digested food products on the intestinal mucosa. Intestinal juice also contains water, salts and mucus. The digestion of the major sources of food (carbohydrate, fat and protein) in the small intestine is dealt with below.

Digestion of carbohydrate

Carbohydrate is present in the diet in several forms – as polysaccharides, disaccharides and monosaccharides. The polysaccharides that can be metabolized are starch (from plants) and glycogen (from animal sources); both these polysaccharides are polymers of glucose. The major polysaccharide is starch and digestion of this begins in the mouth by the enzyme *salivary amylase*. The action of amylase on starch lasts for a very short time, as the food in the mouth is quickly swallowed and, when the food reaches the stomach, gastric acid inactivates the amylase. Once the contents of the stomach have passed into the duodenum the digestion of carbohydrates continues. In the duodenum, *pancreatic amylase* continues to break starch down into smaller polysaccharides and eventually into the disaccharide, maltose. The enterocytes of the villi contain three enzymes: *maltase, lactase* and *sucrase*, which complete the digestion of disaccharides into the monosaccharides glucose, fructose and galactose. All the monosaccharides are subsequently absorbed in the small intestine, from which they will enter the bloodstream and can be metabolized in the body.

Digestion of fats

Fats are not digested in the mouth nor the stomach, through which they pass as fat globules. The process of fat digestion begins in the duodenum where the physical properties of the fats are changed by the emulsifying action of bile. This breaks down the globules and increases the surface area of fat which can come in contact with the pancreatic enzyme *lipase*. Fats are broken down into fatty acids and glycerol, which are absorbed in the small intestine.

Within the cells of the small intestine fat is re-made and formed into small particles, with protein called *chylomicrons*, and these are absorbed into the central lacteal of the villi and eventually taken into the bloodstream.

Digestion of proteins

No digestion of protein takes place in the mouth. In the stomach, the action of hydrochloric acid, present in gastric juice, changes the physical properties of the protein, making it easier to digest. Protein digestion commences in the stomach under the action of the enzyme *pepsin*. Pepsin is produced by the activation of inactive *pepsinogen* by the action of hydrochloric acid (HCl). Proteins are broken down by pepsin to smaller fragments called *peptides*. The process of protein digestion continues in the duodenum with the action of the pancreatic enzymes *trypsin* and *chymotrypsin*. Both these enzymes are produced by the pancreas in inactive forms, *trypsinogen* and *chymotrypsinogen*, which are activated by the alkaline nature of pancreatic juice, which also acts to inactivate the action of pepsin. Within the small intestine enterocytes there are further intestinal enzymes which complete the digestion of protein down to its constituent amino acids. Amino acids are absorbed from the small intestine directly into the bloodstream, from which they are delivered to tissues for metabolism.

Absorption

The absorption of nutrients takes place almost entirely through the villi in the small intestine. Each day, approximately 8–9 litres of water and 1 kg of nutrients pass from the intestinal lumen, across the wall of the intestine and into its blood supply. Proteins, in the form of amino acids, and carbohydrates, as simple sugars, are absorbed by the intestinal cells and pass into the blood capillaries, being carried by the portal vein to the liver. Fats, in the form of fatty acids and glycerol, are absorbed by the central lacteal of the villi and eventually enter the bloodstream via the lymph.

Peritoneum

Most of the small intestine is attached to the posterior abdominal wall by a double fold of serous membrane called *peritoneum*. The part that lines the abdominal wall is named the *parietal portion* of the peritoneum; the part

Gluten-sensitive enteropathy (coeliac disease) is an immunological disorder characterized by a reaction of the intestinal mucosa, particularly in the jejunum, to gliandin (a component of the gluten of wheat). The intestinal mucosa is damaged, resulting in decreased stimulation of pancreatic hormones, impaired absorption of water and electrolytes and excretion of unabsorbed fats. Symptoms include diarrhoea, steatorrhoea, weight loss and abdominal distension. Coeliac disease is managed by a gluten-free diet (i.e. wheat, rye, barley and oats are avoided).

that is reflected over the organs is called the *visceral portion*. The two layers are in contact with each other but the potential space between them is named the *peritoneal cavity*. The peritoneum has several functions:

- to prevent friction as the abdominal organs move on one another and against the abdominal wall
- to attach the abdominal organs to the abdominal wall (except the duodenum and pancreas which lie behind it)
- to carry blood vessels, lymphatics and nerves to the organs
- to fight infection, as the peritoneum contains many lymphatic nodes.

LARGE INTESTINE

In humans the large intestine is about 1.5 metres long and extends from the end of the ileum to the anus. Apart from the stomach, it is the widest part of the gastrointestinal tract, with a diameter of 5–6 cms. It consists of the caecum, appendix, colon and rectum.

The caecum

The *caecum* is a blind-ending pouch about 7 cm long, entered via the ileo-caecal valve and leading into the colon. Each day about one litre of chyme is released into the caecum. The ileo-caecal valve is a sphincter which prevents the caecal contents passing back into the ileum.

The appendix

The *appendix* is a veriform (worm-like) blind-ending sac projecting from the end of the caecum, and about the size of an adult's little finger. The appendix has no known physiological function in humans, but as a clinical application it is a common site for inflammation (appendicitis).

The colon

The *colon* is the dilated area of the large bowel and it is anatomically divided into several regions (Fig. 7.11).

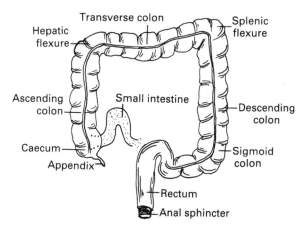

Fig. 7.11 The colon.

Many herbs can aid digestion. For example, *aloe vera* acts as a 'demulcent', coating, lining and protecting the mucous membranes that line the upper part of the digestive tract; it is also a laxative. Many of the essential oils are said to be beneficial to the digestive system. For example, *ginger root* soothes the system; *peppermint* can aid digestion, and is a component of many indigestion and heartburn remedies. It is also used in the management of irritable bowel syndrome. Some of the essential oils such as *orange* and *clove* are digestive stimulants – even inhalation of their vapours can increase the amount of saliva produced.

■ BOX 7.10 Inflammatory bowel disorders

Inflammatory bowel disease (IBD) is the term used to designate the two inflammatory gastrointestinal conditions of Crohn's disease and ulcerative colitis. The distinction between these conditions is not entirely clear, nor is the cause of these disorders. Patients with IBD will experience recurrent bouts of diarrhoea, abdominal pain, lethargy and concomitant weight loss. These disorders are chronic and present in a remitting and relapsing nature.

The *ascending colon* is about 15 cm in length and is much narrower than the caecum. It ascends the right side of the abdomen to the underside of the liver, where it bends forward and to the left at the right colic flexure. The *transverse colon* is about 50 cm in length and it passes across the abdomen underneath the spleen; it curves sharply downward at the left colic flexure. The *descending colon* is about 25 cm in length and it passes down the left side of the abdomen to become the sigmoid colon. The rectum is continuous with the *sigmoid colon*.

The material that enters into the large intestine consists of water, salt, very little food material, roughage, which is indigestible, and bacteria.

Movements of the colon are similar to those seen in the small intestine, involving a strong non-propulsive muscular movement, segmentation. Peristalsis also occurs in the colon, propelling faeces towards the rectum.

The rectum

The *rectum* is a muscular tube about 12–15 cm long, capable of great distension. It usually remains empty until just before defaecation. Mass movement within colon leads to a sudden distension of the rectal walls, this is termed the 'call to stool', when an individual becomes aware of the need to defaecate.

The rectum opens to the exterior via the *anal canal*, which is about 4 cm long. The anal canal has two sphincter muscles: the internal one is controlled by the autonomic nervous system and the external anal sphincter is under voluntary control.

Defaecation is a reflex contraction in response to faeces entering the rectum. This distension causes a reflex contraction of the rectal muscles which tend to expel the contents through the anus. This reflex is controlled by the relaxation or contraction of the external anal sphincter.

■ BOX 7.11 Haemorrhoids

Haemorrhoids are the enlargement or inflammation of the haemorrhoid veins, which supply the anal canal. Haemorrhoids cause pain, itching and bleeding around the anus. Treatment includes the use of hydrocortisone creams and suppositories or, in extreme cases, surgery.

■ BOX 7.12 Constipation

Constipation refers to the difficult passage of hard stools. Constipation is therefore the opposite of diarrhoea in that food residues become hard, due to the reabsorption of water when they remain in the colon for a prolonged period of time. They may become difficult and often painful to eliminate. Constipation often occurs when a diet contains insufficient fibre. Food residues tend to remain in the colon until eventually both the colon and rectum are full of faecal material. The constipation sufferer can complain of abdominal pain and abdominal distension or bloatedness. The most common causes of constipation are listed below;

- dehydration (decrease in fluid intake/increase of fluid loss)
- drugs (certain analgesics and antihypertensives may lead to constipation)
- inactivity (exercise tends to stimulate motility)
- insufficient dietary fibre
- depression and dementia.

There are many other causes of constipation, including avoidance of defaecation, e.g. the embarrassment of a patient having to use a bedpan or commode in the close vicinity of other patients. It is important to be aware of the patient who has mobility difficulties, who may also avoid defaecation as they cannot move to the toilet. In general, constipation should be treated by improvement in diet, increasing fluid intake, taking plenty of exercise and developing a regular bowel habit. In extreme cases it may be necessary to resort to drugs to correct constipation. These drugs are called laxatives or aperients, and they work by either increasing motility of the intestine or by drawing fluid back from the wall of the colon to make faeces more fluid. Other aperients act as lubricants.

Functions of the large intestine

The large intestine has several major functions:

- storage of food residues prior to their elimination
- absorption of water, electrolytes and vitamins
- synthesis of vitamin K and vitamin B_{12} by colonic bacteria
- secretion of mucus to lubricate faeces
- elimination of food residue as faeces.

One function of the colon is to store unabsorbed and unused food residues, 70% of which is eliminated within 72 hours, the remaining 30% can remain in the bowel for up to a week or longer. The amount of water reabsorbed from colonic contents depends upon the length of time food residue remains in the colon. In a constipated individual, the food residue can remain in the colon for several days, during which time the more and more water is reabsorbed, this can result in hard pellets of faeces which may be difficult to eliminate (see Box 7.12). Many bacteria (mainly anaerobes) inhabit the large intestine and exhibit a symbiotic relationship in

Massage can be specifically applied to the large intestine to improve elimination. Abdominal massage can also stimulate peristalsis, relieving intestinal gas and colic. However, contraindications to abdominal massage include inflammatory bowel diseases, and medical advice should always be sought.

■ **BOX 7.13 Diarrhoea**

Diarrhoea results when movements of the intestine occur too rapidly for water to be absorbed in the colon. Stools are therefore produced in large amounts, and may range from being loose to being entirely liquid. Diarrhoea, depending on its severity and duration, can be a nuisance or can be fatal. If diarrhoea is severe, large amounts of fluid may be lost from the body, resulting in dehydration and electrolyte (i.e. sodium and potassium) imbalance. The following are potential causes of diarrhoea:

- diet (highly seasoned food/food allergies)
- irritable bowel syndrome/diverticular disease
- drugs (antibiotics, iron preparations and laxatives can all result in diarrhoea)
- infections (organisms can cause intestinal infection)
- inflammatory bowel conditions (Crohn's disease/ulcerative colitis)
- malabsorptive disorder of the bowel (coeliac disease – gluten-sensitive enteritis)
- stress (diarrhoea may be a physiological response to stress).

In the management of diarrhoea, the predisposing cause should be sought and treated, and dehydration and electrolyte imbalances must be corrected.

humans; that is, each derives mutual benefit from one another and they live together harmoniously. It is important to be aware that although these bacteria are harmless in the intestine, they can become pathogenic if introduced into another part of the body.

THE LIVER, BILIARY SYSTEM AND PANCREAS

The liver

The liver is the largest organ in the body, weighing on average 1.5 kg in men and 1.3 kg in women. It is situated in the upper right of the abdominal cavity. Anatomically the liver consists of four lobes, the largest being the *right lobe* which lies over the right colic flexure and right kidney. The smaller *left lobe* lies directly over the stomach; the two lesser segments of the right lobe are *caudate* and *quadrate* lobes, these are located on the underside of the liver. The ligament which attaches the liver to the abdominal wall is known as the faliciform ligament.

The blood supply to the liver is unique in that it is delivered by two sources. The *hepatic portal vein* drains the digestive tract, whilst the *hepatic artery* supplies blood rich in oxygen from the arterial system (Fig. 7.12).

Structurally the liver is divided into a large number of *lobules*, each of which measures 1–2 mm in diameter. These constitute the functional units of the liver. Lobules are hexagonal in shape and consist of a central vein from which single columns of liver cells, hepatocytes, radiate (Fig. 7.13).

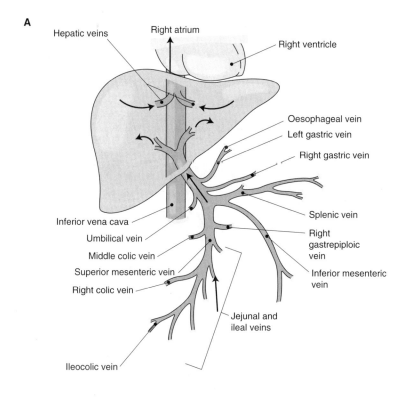

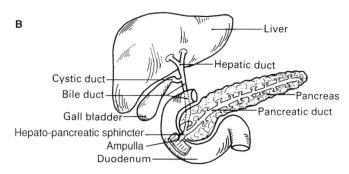

Fig. 7.12 (A) The hepatic portal venous system (from Cheshire E. Crash course: gastrointestinal system. London: Mosby–Wolfe; 1997); (B) pancreas, gall bladder and liver.

Between the layers of cells lie *sinusoids*, which receive blood from both artery and vein and drain into a central vein. The sinusoids contain *Kupffer cells*, which are phagocytic in nature and provide a defence mechanism in the liver. Surrounding liver cells, and in direct contact with them, is a network of minute tubules called *bile canaliculi*, which carry bile produced within the liver cells.

The liver is an organ which is vital to life. It is metabolically very active in the synthesis and catabolism (breakdown) of carbohydrates, fats, proteins and vitamins. It also metabolizes and detoxifies hormones, steroids and other substances, such as drugs and alcohol. The main functions of the liver are:

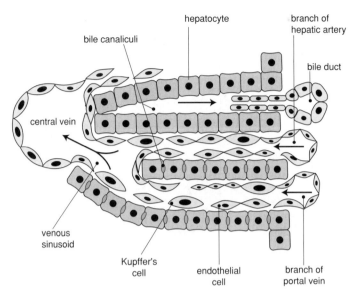

Fig. 7.13 General features of a liver lobule (from Cheshire E. Crash course: gastrointestinal system. London: Mosby–Wolfe; 1997).

1. Metabolic

- stored fat is broken down to provide energy
- excess amino acids are broken down and converted to urea
- drugs and poisons are detoxified
- vitamin A is synthesized from carotene
- plasma proteins (albumin and globulin) are synthesized
- excess carbohydrate is converted to fat for storage in adipose tissue
- prothrombin and fibrinogen are synthesized from amino acids
- antibodies and antitoxins are manufactured
- heparin is manufactured.

2. Storage functions

- vitamins A and D
- anti-anaemic factor
- iron from the diet and from worn-out red blood cells
- glucose is stored as glycogen.

3. Secretory functions

- bile is formed from constituents brought by the blood.

The biliary system

The biliary system removes waste products from the liver and carries bile to the duodenum to aid digestion. Several elements compose the biliary system (Fig. 7.14):

- right and left hepatic ducts, which unite to form the common hepatic duct
- the gall bladder, which acts as a reservoir for bile

■ BOX 7.14 **Cirrhosis of the liver**

Cirrhosis of the liver involves the death of hepatocytes and their replacement by fibrous connective tissue. The liver becomes pale in colour due to the presence of excess white connective tissue. It also becomes firmer and the surface becomes nodular. The loss of hepatocytes impairs the function of the liver; this can result in jaundice, and the build-up of connective tissue can impede blood flow through the liver. Cirrhosis frequently develops in alcohol abusers and may also occur as a result of biliary obstruction, hepatitis or nutritional deficiencies. Under most conditions mature hepatocytes can proliferate and regenerate the liver's functional capacity. However, if the liver is severely damaged, the hepatocytes may be unable to regenerate and liver transplantation may be indicated.

- the cystic duct, leading from the gall bladder
- the bile duct, formed by the junction of the common hepatic and cystic ducts.

The *gall bladder* is a pear-shaped organ, situated on the undersurface of the right lobe of the liver. Its main function is to act as a reservoir for bile. The capacity of the gall bladder is between 30 and 60 ml, but because of its ability to absorb water the bile it contains becomes increasingly concentrated. When fatty foods enter the duodenum from the stomach, the sphincter at the entrance of the bile duct relaxes and the bile stored in the gall bladder is driven into the intestine by contraction of the muscular walls of the gall bladder. Substances that bring about the contraction of the gall bladder are referred to as cholagogues. The secretion of bile is under the influence of both hormonal and nervous stimuli. The major hormonal stimulus for bile release is the hormone *cholecystokinin* (CCK).

Bile

Bile is a thick, greenish-yellow fluid secreted by liver cells. The liver secretes, on average, about 0.5–1.0 litre of bile per day. Bile is mainly a water secretion (97%); other components include bile salts, bile pigments, cholesterol, mucus and a variety of ions. Bile is similar to pancreatic juice, with a slightly alkaline pH of 7.8–8.0. The main function of bile in digestion lies in its role in the emulsification of fats and the consequent absorption of lipids, fat-soluble vitamins and iron.

■ BOX 7.15 **Gallstones**

Cholesterol, or other deposits of the constituents of bile, may precipitate in the gall bladder to produce gallstones. Occasionally a gallstone can pass out of the gall bladder and enter the cystic duct, blocking the release of bile. Such a condition is very painful and can interfere with normal digestion. In many instances these gallstones must be removed endoscopically or surgically.

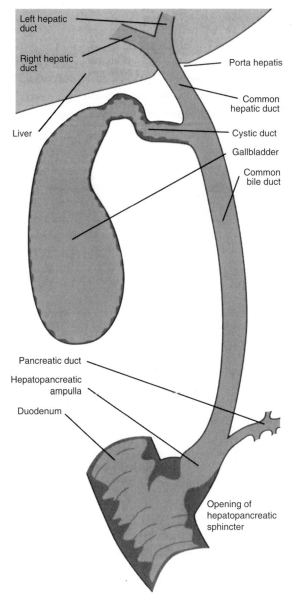

Fig. 7.14 The gall bladder and its ducts (from Hinchcliff SM, Montague SE, Watson R. Physiology for nursing practice. London: Ballière Tindall; 1996).

The pancreas

The *pancreas* is a gland with both endocrine and exocrine functions, it is therefore described as a mixed gland. Structurally, the pancreas is a soft, greyish-pink gland, 12–15 cm long. The head of the pancreas lies in the curve of the duodenum, the body lies behind the stomach and the tail extends as far as the spleen. The pancreatic duct lies within the organ (Fig. 7.15)

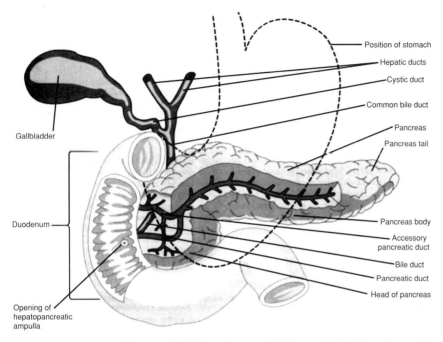

Fig. 7.15 The pancreas (from Hinchcliff SM, Montague SE, Watson R. Physiology for nursing practice. London: Ballière Tindall; 1996).

The cells of the *islets of Langerhans* make up the endocrine part of the pancreas, they secrete hormones which pass directly into the bloodstream (see Chs 9 and 12). The exocrine pancreas has a major role to play in digestion. The digestive function is served by *acinar cells*, which resemble structurally the cells of the salivary glands. These cells form and store *zymogen granules* which consist of inactive enzymes (proenzymes: pancreatic trypsinogen, pancreatic amylase and pancreatic lipase). These enzymes are discharged in response to stimulation, mainly hormonal, and they are secreted into the pancreatic duct. About 1.5 litres of pancreatic juice is secreted a day; the bulk being sodium- and bicarbonate-rich fluid, which neutralizes acid entering the duodenum from the stomach.

■ **BOX 7.16 Pancreatitis**

Pancreatitis is an inflammation of the pancreas, occurring quite commonly. It may result from alcohol abuse, use of certain drugs, pancreatic duct blockage and pancreatic cancer. Symptoms can range from mild abdominal pain to systemic shock.

METABOLISM

Metabolism is the term used to describe the complex process by which food is converted to heat and energy. Metabolism is composed of two processes: anabolism and catabolism, which work simultaneously to build up and break down molecules, respectively. All the energy-using processes of the body, such as digestion, are dependent upon metabolism, as they are synthetic processes whereby large molecules, such as proteins, are made for use in muscle and other tissue.

The amount of food we require in 24 hours varies with age, size, sex and activity. The amount of energy each food substance gives is measured in kilojoules (kJ) and the amount of heat given off is measured in kilocalories (kcal). A kilocalorie is the amount of heat required to raise the temperature of 1 kg of water through 1°C.

DIGESTIVE SYSTEM QUESTIONS

Diagrams—Questions 325–349

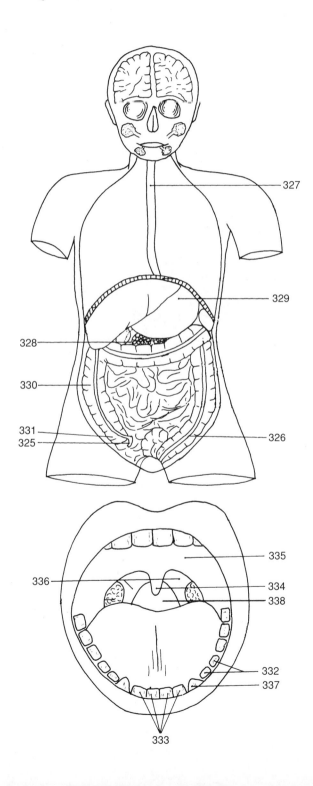

325–331. Digestive tract

A. Oesophagus
B. Stomach
C. Ascending colon
D. Duodenum
E. Caecum
F. Appendix
G. Pelvic colon

325
326
327
328
329
330
331

332–338. Mouth and teeth

A. Fauces
B. Oropharynx
C. Uvula
D. Palate
E. Premolars
F. Canine
G. Incisors

332
333
334
335
336
337
338

339–343. Stomach

A. Greater curvature
B. Fundus
C. Pylorus
D. Cardiac orifice
E. Pyloric sphincter

| 339
| 340
| 341
| 342
| 343

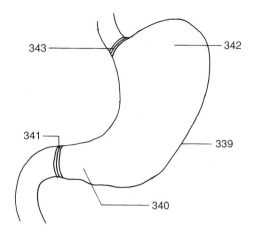

344–349. The liver, pancreas and duodenum

A. Cystic duct
B. Hepato-pancre-
   atic sphincter
C. Right hepatic
   duct
D. Bile duct
E. Pancreatic duct
F. Gall bladder

| 344
| 345
| 346
| 347
| 348
| 349

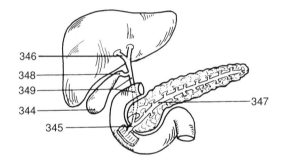

Questions 350–357 are of the multiple choice type

350. **Which one of the following carbohydrates is acted on by the enzyme salivary amylase?**   350
   A. Lactose
   B. Maltose
   C. Sucrose
   D. Starch.

351. **The amount of water in the cells of the body is approximately:**   351
   A. 45 litres
   B. 30 litres
   C. 15 litres
   D. 5 litres.

352. **Which one of the following organs is not a part of the digestive system?**   352
   A. Liver
   B. Oesophagus
   C. Pharynx
   D. Spleen.

353. **In the human mouth there are:**   353
   A. 36 permanent teeth
   B. 20 temporary teeth
   C. 4 incisors
   D. 8 canines.

354. **The tongue:**   354
   A. is attached to the maxilla
   B. is attached to the hyoid bone
   C. is covered with ciliated mucous membrane
   D. contains many taste buds on its inferior surface.

355. **Which one of the following is not a salivary gland?**   355
   A. Parotid
   B. Pineal
   C. Submandibular
   D. Sublingual.

356. **The oesophagus:**   356
   A. is approximately 30 cm long
   B. lies in front of the trachea
   C. lies behind the aorta
   D. extends from the pharynx to the stomach.

357. **To which one of the following parts of the intestine is the appendix attached?**   357
   A. Caecum
   B. Duodenum
   C. Ileum
   D. Sigmoid colon.

Questions 358–377 are of the true/false type   T | F

358–361. Of the essential food substances:
    358. carbohydrate provides energy
    359. fats transport vitamins C and B
    360. minerals are necessary for fluid balance
    361. protein is necessary for the formation of blood.

362–365. Protein:
    362. can be used for heat and energy
    363. can be changed into urea in the kidneys
    364. is absorbed in the form of amino acids
    365. is necessary for the growth of tissue.

366–369. Glucose:
    366. can be stored unaltered in the liver
    367. if taken in excess can be stored as fat
    368. is one end product of the digestion of carbohydrate
    369. helps to maintain the body temperature.

370–373. The portal vein carries:
    370. bile to the liver
    371. glucose to the liver
    372. most of the fat to the liver
    373. iron to the liver.

374–377. The villi:
    374. contain blood vessels but no lymphatic vessels
    375. are only present in the jejunum
    376. absorb the end products of digestion
    377. attaches the bowel to the abdominal wall.

Questions 378–388 are of the matching items type

378–379. **From the list on the left select the statement which describes each substance on the right.**
A. Is an enzyme	378. Antianaemic factor	378
B. Is the chemical name for vitamin E	379. Ergosterol.	379
C. Is present in outer leaves of cabbage		
D. Is a fatty substance in the skin		
E. Is secreted by the walls of the stomach		

380–382. **From the list on the left pair the organs with the functions on the right.**
A. Stomach	380. Absorption	380
B. Small intestine	381. Elimination	381
C. Colon	382. Ingestion.	382
D. Oesophagus		
E. Mouth		

383–384. **From the list on the left select a function for each organ listed on the right.**
A. Secretes bile	383. Pancreas	383
B. Secretes amylase	384. Stomach.	384
C. Secretes maltose		
D. Secretes sucrase		
E. Secretes pepsin		

385–386. **From the list on the left select the statement which describes each substance on the right.**
A. Is acid in the stomach	385. Bolus	385
B. Is coloured by bile	386. Faeces.	386
C. Is a digestive enzyme		
D. Is masticated food		
E. Is a secretion of the pancreas		

387–388. **From the list on the left select the statement which describes each word on the right.**
A. Is milk sugar	387. Lacteal	387
B. Is a lymphatic vessel	388. Lactase.	388
C. Is part of the stomach		
D. Is a carbohydrate enzyme		
E. Is part of the liver		

The skin

■ KEY POINTS

- The integumentary system
- The functions of the integumentary system
- The epidermis
- The dermis
- The hair, nails and glands
- Touch.

THE INTEGUMENTARY SYSTEM

The skin, hair, nails and glands make up the *integumentary system*. The name comes from the Latin *integumentum*, which means a *covering*.

The skin

The skin is the largest, the heaviest and one of the most active organs – an adult's skin has a surface area of around 1.5 to 2 square metres. It is a boundary or barrier between the individual and the external environment. The appearance of the skin can reveal much about a person. It is an indicator of general health, age and physiological state, and also the emotions.

The skin has many functions – it is protective, it excretes waste products, it regulates body temperature and it is an important sensory organ.

Many factors influence the health of the skin; these include nutrition, circulation, and the use of drugs, the environment and hygiene. Of all the organs of the body, the skin is the most exposed to and at risk from injury. A wide range of substances with which it comes into contact – clothing, metals, soaps, detergents, foods, animals, plants, drugs – will affect it.

Healthy skin is clear, an even colour, soft, supple to touch, moist and unblemished, with a good degree of elasticity. However, genetic factors and the ageing process, and other factors such as smoking, overexposure to sunlight, poor diet, lack of sleep, etc. will influence the appearance and texture of the skin. The skin can become dehydrated, dry or oily, or develop eruptions, and may develop sensitivity to extremes of weather or temperature. It can be affected by allergic reactions – rashes can appear, or the skin may become irritated and inflamed.

The general condition of the skin must be observed for dehydration, presence of pressure sores, rashes or other skin conditions, for example. When caring for the skin, the individual's preferences and cultural/religious needs must be adhered to. In general, the skin requires to be washed, well rinsed and thoroughly dried. Some soaps can alter the skin's pH and their use should be avoided. If possible, a shower should be taken in preference to a bath as there is less of a cross-infection risk. Any changes that are observed on the skin should be reported and acted upon.

Structure

The skin consists of an outer layer of stratified squamous epithelium called the *epidermis* and an inner layer of elastic fibrous connective tissue called the *dermis*. Underneath this lies the *subcutaneous layer*, which consists of primarily adipose tissue. This attaches to underlying tissues – the *superficial fascia* that covers muscle and bone.

■ **BOX 8.1 Fingerprints**

The dermal papillae appear on the surface of the skin as markings. On the fingertips these patterns are the fingerprints, which are different in every individual and are, therefore, so useful for purposes of identification.

The epidermis is attached to the dermis by interlocking projections – *epidermal ridges* extend downwards into the dermis, and *dermal papillae* extend upwards into the epidermis. Fibres in the dermis extend into the subcutaneous layer, so that the skin is attached securely to the tissues.

THE FUNCTIONS OF THE INTEGUMENTARY SYSTEM

The main functions of the integumentary system are:

- protection
- regulation of body temperature
- elimination of waste
- sensation
- manufacture of vitamin D.

Protection

The skin, hair and nails, and glands have important protective roles, including:

- protection of internal parts of the body from injury such as physical abrasion
- protection from chemical agents
- prevention of water loss – dehydration
- protection from UV light
- prevention of the entry of microorganisms, which could potentially cause disease.

Regulation of body temperature

A temperature-regulating centre in the brain controls the temperature of the body. The skin acts as a thermostat, keeping the temperature of the body between 36 and 37°C. Various physiological activities generate heat, including muscle contraction. The digestive organs, the liver in particular, contribute to heat production. Heat is lost from the body in urine, faeces and expired air, but mostly by *sweating*.

When you become hot, the arterioles in the dermis dilate, bringing more blood to the capillaries in the skin. The skin becomes red and hot; heat is

■ **BOX 8.2 Febrile conditions**

In febrile (fever) conditions, the control centre in the brain is upset, and if the body temperature rises above 39°C, some attempt must be made to lower it. Tepid sponging, or covering the patient in a cold, wet sheet, and exposing to an electric fan to speed up the rate of evaporation, may lower the temperature.

■ BOX 8.3 Hypothermia

Hypothermia is a condition where the body temperature is below 35°C. If the temperature falls below this, the temperature control mechanisms fail, the muscles contract, vasoconstriction does not occur, the blood pressure drops and the heart rate falls. If the temperature falls below 25 degrees centigrade, death is likely. The very young and the elderly are more prone to hypothermia.

lost by radiation and conduction. At the same time, the sweat glands produce more sweat, which will evaporate because of the heat in the skin and circulating air. If the air is circulating rapidly, evaporation will occur at a faster rate and consequently the heat loss will be greater.

In cold conditions, when the air temperature is below body temperature, the arterioles in the dermis constrict. Less blood circulates in the dermis, which appears white and cold, and less heat is lost to the cold air. The sweat glands become less active, and shivering may occur. Shivering is an attempt to balance the heat loss when there is danger of body temperature falling below normal.

Elimination of waste

The skin is also an organ of elimination. Salts, lactic acid, urea and other metabolic wastes are eliminated from the body in sweat.

Sensation

The skin is the chief agent of communication between the external environment and the body. The skin contains numerous nerve endings that convey the sensations of *touch, temperature, pressure* and *pain* to the brain.

Manufacture of vitamin D

Modified cholesterol molecules (precursor molecules) are found in the deepest part of the epidermis. The ultraviolet (UV) rays in sunlight convert this into vitamin D. Very little sunlight is required for this process. Vitamin D is an important vitamin – it is necessary for the absorption of calcium and phosphorus from food.

■ BOX 8.4 Absorption

The skin has the ability to absorb some substances, including the essential oils that are central to the practice of aromatherapy.

Substances that can be absorbed by the skin and gain entry to the body include fat-soluble substances such as steroids and the fat-soluble vitamins A, D and E, and oxygen and carbon dioxide. Harmful organic solvents such as paint thinners, and salts of heavy metals such as lead, mercury and nickel can also be absorbed.

The use of therapeutic *transdermal patches* and topical medication is becoming widespread, e.g. hormone replacement medication, analgesic medication in the form of creams and gels, and also nicotine to aid those giving up smoking.

■ BOX 8.5 Callosities

If the epidermis is subjected to intermittent pressure and friction, it will thicken and become hard and scaly. These areas are called callosities. They occur most commonly on the soles of the feet, and on the hands of those who repeatedly use tools of instruments that cause pressure and friction.

The precise areas where thickened skin and callosities appear on the feet is considered significant in reflexology practice, as they are thought to indicate organs or systems where imbalance or dysfunction may manifest.

THE EPIDERMIS

The epidermis has a protective function. It appears thicker in some areas than in others. For example, the thickest areas of epidermis are on the soles of the feet and the palms of the hands – areas subject to wear and tear, pressure and friction.

The epidermis consists of layers (*strata*) of closely packed cells. The upper cells are dead, their cytoplasm having been replaced by a tough fibrous material called *keratin*. The cytoskeleton of skin cells is composed of keratin, a protein that acts as a strengthening, protective and waterproofing agent for the skin. The upper layers are continually shed, being replaced by cells from the deeper layers – the *germinative* layers. The average life of an epidermal cell is between 21 and 27 days. Normally, the entire epidermis is replaced every 40 days.

The epidermis does not have a blood supply or nerves. All oxygen and nutrients reach the epidermis by diffusion from the dermis. This is why the superficial cells die off – they are too far from the source of oxygen and nutrients in the blood.

Structure of the epidermis

There are typically four layers of cells. However, in areas that are subject to friction, there may be five (Fig. 8.1)

1. *Stratum corneum* – the outermost layer, which consists of layers of tightly packed, flat, dead cells. These cells have become fully *keratinized*.
2. *Stratum lucidum* – lies under the stratum corneum. It is more apparent in areas of thicker epidermis. Here, the cells are also flat and dead, but they are clear in appearance.
3. *Stratum granulosum* – this is a thin layer of cells where there are granules of a material called *keratohyalin*. It is an intermediate layer, where the nuclei of the cells begin to degrade, and the process of keratinization begins.
4. *Stratum spinosum* – this is called the 'prickly layer', as its cells (*keratinocytes*) possess interlocking cytoplasmic processes, which act as

■ BOX 8.6 Repair

If the epidermis is burned or damaged it can repair itself. This does not occur in the dermis. A deep burn involving both the epidermis and the dermis requires a *skin graft* before it will heal.

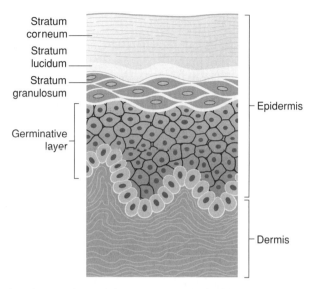

Stratum corneum

Stratum lucidum

Stratum granulosum

Germinative layer

Epidermis

Dermis

Fig. 8.1 The skin, showing the main layers of the epidermis (from Waugh A, Grant A. Ross and Wilson Anatomy and physiology in health and illness. 9th edn. Edinburgh: Churchill Livingstone; 2001).

anchoring junctions. These bond the deepest layer of the epidermis to the stratum granulosum.

5. *Stratum germinativum* – this is known as the basal layer, the deepest layer of the epidermis. Its cells lie close to the dermis, from where it receives its blood supply. It is here that new cells are formed; these eventually become the upper layers. Cells called *melanocytes* produce the pigment that gives skin and hair its colour – *melanin*. In the basal layer, nerve endings called *Merkel's discs* (or tactile discs) give the skin its sense of touch.

■ BOX 8.7 Skin pigmentation

Exposure to the sun's rays increases the amount of pigment produced in the epidermis, and this in turn protects the deeper layers of the skin from damage by the sun. Freckles and moles are small areas where melanin pigment is concentrated. A genetic condition called *albinism*, where the skin and hair are white, and the iris of the eye is pink, occurs when an individual does not produce melanin. *Vitiligo* is the name given to a condition where there is partial or total loss of skin pigmentation. Some of the hormones produced in pregnancy can stimulate melanin synthesis, resulting in a darkening of facial skin – the 'mask of pregnancy' or *chloasma*.

Melanoma is a malignant tumour of melanocytes. This condition is increasing in all fair-skinned populations, worldwide. Exposure to sunlight, especially in childhood, is a significant factor.

■ **BOX 8.8 Skin ageing**

The skin is constantly ageing, but the effects are not usually noticeable until the late 40s. The numbers of fibroblasts decreases; this means that collagen synthesis decreases. In addition, the collagen fibres decrease in number, become stiffer and then break apart. Elastin fibres thicken and form clumps, losing elasticity. The result is wrinkles, folds and loss of firmness in the skin.

THE DERMIS

The dermis is the inner part of the skin. It is firmly anchored to the epidermis by the dermal papillae. It is composed of fibrous connective tissue, with bundles of collagen and elastin fibres that provide support, elasticity and resilience. Unlike the epidermis, the dermis has a blood and a nerve supply – there is a vast network of blood and lymphatic capillaries, and nerve endings (Fig. 8.2).

Structure of the dermis

1. The more superficial part of the dermis is known as the *papillary region* because of the projecting dermal papillae. It is mainly composed of fine bundles of collagen fibres. Nerve endings, which detect different types of touch and sensation, are present here. These are called *Meissner's* and *Pacini's corpuscles*.
2. Lying below the papillary region is the *reticular layer*. This is composed of interlaced bundles of collagen fibres and coarser elastin fibres. The structure allows the skin to be moved about in many directions.

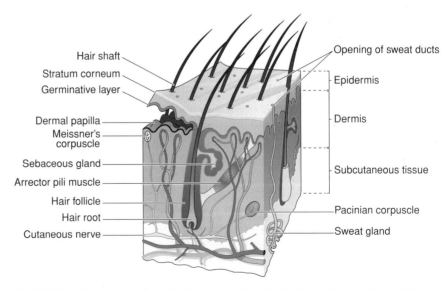

Fig. 8.2 The skin, showing the main structures in the dermis (from Waugh A, Grant A. Ross and Wilson Anatomy and physiology in health and illness. 9th edn. Edinburgh: Churchill Livingstone; 2001).

■ BOX 8.9 Stretch marks

Silver white stretch marks, or *striae*, are the result of overstretching of the collagen and elastin fibres during pregnancy or weight gain.

■ BOX 8.10 Pressure sores

Unrelieved pressure, such as that caused by sitting or lying in the same position for long periods, occludes the capillaries. The cells or the dermis are deprived of their blood supply, and some of them will die. This can be the beginning of a pressure sore, and it may be present even if the epidermis appears healthy.

Pressure sores are areas of damage to the skin and also, usually, to the underlying tissues. They can be caused by direct pressure, shearing forces and friction. The extent of the damage can vary from a superficial redness of the skin to a deep ulceration involving muscle and even bone. Early identification of people at risk is of paramount importance as steps can then be taken to prevent pressure sore occurrence. Various assessment tools are in current use.

THE HAIR, NAILS AND GLANDS

The hair, nails, sweat glands and sebaceous glands are described as *appendages* of the skin, and form part of the integumentary system.

Hair

Hair is derived from the same tissue as the epidermis. The only parts of the skin that do not have hair are the palms of the hands and soles of the feet. Hair is protective in function, for example hair on the head protects the skin from sunlight, and eyebrows and lashes protect the eyes. Hair also helps to keep us warm.

Hair is made of very closely packed keratinized cells. In each hair shaft there are three concentric layers of cells – a central *medulla*, a *cortex* and an outer *cuticle*. Hair grows out from a *follicle* in the dermis.

Attached to the hair follicles are small involuntary muscles, the *arrectores pilorum*. When these muscles contract, they cause the hair to 'stand on end'. This is usually a response to emotion, especially fear. The body becomes more alert and sensitive to changes in the environment, such as air pressure, movement and temperature. The arrectores pilorum will also contract in cold conditions, when the phenomenon is known as 'goose bumps'. The contraction of these muscles, and shivering, generates heat.

Nails

In humans, nails protect the very sensitive tips of the fingers and toes. The nail *matrix*, directly below the cuticle, is the only part that grows; it has nerves and blood vessels. The visible part of the nail, the nail *plate*, consists of very tightly packed keratinized cells.

Sebaceous glands

Near the root of each hair is a small saccular exocrine gland. This is the sebaceous gland, which produces an oily substance called *sebum*. Sebum consists of a mixture of fats, cholesterol, proteins and inorganic salts. This acts as a lubricant for the hair, preventing it from drying and becoming brittle; it also helps prevent evaporation of water from the skin. It softens the skin and protects it from infection, as it is mildly antiseptic. However,

■ BOX 8.11 Sebaceous glands

Oversecretion of sebum, due to the influence of certain hormones, such as the androgens, can result in blocked oil glands. A 'whitehead' forms; if the sebum dries out it becomes discoloured and a 'blackhead' results. Acne is an inflammation of the sebaceous glands, often associated with the increase in sebum production at puberty. The hair follicles are colonized by bacteria, epithelium grows over the follicles – this is often called 'blocked pores'. The retention of sebum and bacterial proliferation results in inflammation and eruptions.

millions of microorganisms adhere to it, therefore care must be taken to swab the skin with antiseptic or remove the sebum prior to penetration by a needle or scalpel.

Sweat glands

Sweat glands (sudoriferous glands) are found on most areas of the skin, but many are located in the palms of the hands, the soles of the feet and the forehead. These glands are coiled tubular structures, with ducts that open onto the surface of the epidermis at pores. Sweat is a watery fluid containing electrolytes and some waste substances. It is continually being excreted and evaporated into the surrounding air.

There are two types of sweat glands, eccrine and apocrine.

1. Eccrine glands are responsible for sweating during physical exertion or emotional stress. Therefore, their function is to cool the body, and eliminate small amounts of waste materials in the sweat, which is 99% water.
2. Apocrine glands are less numerous, and are located in the hairy parts of the axillary and anogenital regions. Their secretions have a stronger odour, and are produced as a response to stress, hormones or sexual arousal.

Many complementary therapies, especially massage, aromatherapy and reflexology, involve the use of carefully applied touch and skin contact. In addition to producing a range of physical and physiological effects, these therapies meet a fundamental human need – nurturing through touch.

TOUCH

Specialized receptors are found in the skin, which provide a sensory input to the brain, and convey many impressions of the surroundings. There are nerve receptors that detect light pressure, light touch, heavy touch, deep pressure, continuous pressure, vibrations of various frequencies and skin displacement. Hair follicle receptors detect movement of hairs. Free nerve endings that detect pain are called nociceptors. These can also detect extremes in temperature and the chemicals liberated by injured cells. Therefore, the skin is the major organ of sensation.

The sense of touch is vital to physical and emotional well-being. It is our first means of communication. It is necessary for the stimulation of some physiological processes such as growth. Touch deprivation can lead to emotional and social problems.

THE SKIN QUESTIONS

Diagrams—Questions 389–394

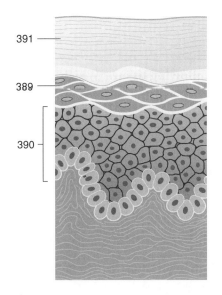

389–394. The skin

A. Stratum corneum
B. Sweat gland duct
C. Sebaceous gland
D. Blood vessel
E. Germinative layer
F. Stratum granulosum

389
390
391
392
393
394

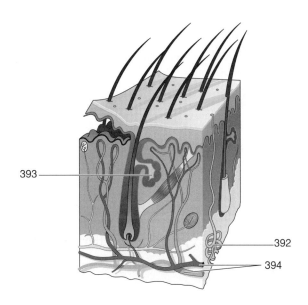

Questions 395–401 are of the multiple choice type

395. Which one of the following is not a function of the skin?   395
  A. The excretion of waste
  B. The manufacture of vitamin A
  C. The regulation of body temperature
  D. It helps to maintain fluid balance.

396. The epidermis is composed of one of the following tissues. Which one?   396
  A. Adipose tissue
  B. Elastic fibrous tissue
  C. Columnar epithelium
  D. Stratified squamous epithelium.

397. Which one of the following statements describes keratin? It is: 397
  A. a type of protoplasm
  B. a tough, fibrous material
  C. the colouring matter in the skin
  D. the precursor of vitamin D.

398. The dermis is composed of one of the following tissues. Which one?   398
  A. Adipose tissue
  B. Epithelial tissue
  C. White fibrous tissue
  D. Muscle tissue.

399. The epidermis contains one of the following: 399
  A. ducts of glands
  B. blood vessels
  C. sebaceous glands
  D. sensory nerve endings.

400. Which one of the following substances is not present in sweat?   400
  A. Calcium
  B. Lactic acid
  C. Urea
  D. Water.

401. Which one of the following statements is true? A patient with a febrile condition: 401
  A. is in no danger if his temperature is below 40°C
  B. will sweat more as his temperature rises
  C. should be treated by tepid sponging
  D. should be given extra blankets.

Questions 402–433 are of the true/false type   T | F

402–405. The dermis contains:
   402. ductless glands
   403. sebaceous glands
   404. lymphatic glands
   405. sweat glands.

406–409. Melanin:
   406. is present in the epidermis
   407. increases on exposure to the rays of the sun
   408. has a protective function
   409. makes the skin waterproof.

410–413. The arterioles in the skin:
   410. dilate when you become hot
   411. constrict in cold conditions
   412. dilate in a cold bath
   413. dilate during exercise.

414–417. The sweat glands are:
   414. simple tubular glands
   415. coiled tubular glands
   416. saccular glands
   417. glands with ducts.

418–421. The excretion of sweat:
   418. is a continuous process
   419. helps to maintain electrolyte balance
   420. cools the body
   421. gets rid of the waste products of protein metabolism.

422–425. Body heat is gained by:
   422. shivering
   423. circulation of air at 30°C
   424. contraction of the arrectores pilorum muscles
   425. constriction of the arterioles.

426–429. Sebum:
   426. acts as a mild antiseptic
   427. is a waste product of metabolism
   428. is a trap for microorganisms
   429. is secreted by the hair follicles.

430–433. The arrectores pilorum muscles contract when the individual is:
   430. exercising
   431. cold
   432. afraid
   433. in pain.

The urinary system

INTRODUCTION

The main function of the kidney is to purify the blood and to rid the body of waste/excess products. It does this by filtering blood and producing *urine*, which contains the waste products to be excreted. Urine is produced by the following three processes:

- glomerular filtration
- selective reabsorption
- tubular secretion.

An explanation of these processes will be given later in the chapter.

The urinary system consists of two kidneys, two ureters, one urinary bladder and one urethra (Fig. 9.1). The functions of the urinary system are:

- to control water and electrolyte balance
- to control the excretion of waste products
- to control acid–base (pH) balance
- to assist in the control of blood pressure
- to produce red blood cells in the event of a sudden loss of blood
- to transport and store urine
- to eliminate urine from the body.

ANATOMY

The *kidneys* are two bean-shaped organs lying on the posterior abdominal wall, one on either side of the first to third lumbar vertebrae. The right kidney is lower than the left, due to the presence of the liver. Each kidney measures approximately $11 \times 7 \times 3$ cm and weighs around 150 g. On the top of each kidney is an adrenal gland, which is part of the endocrine system (see Ch. 12). The kidneys are covered in a capsule and embedded in a pad of fat. The latter serves as protection and insulation. If a kidney is cut longitudinally, it will appear to consist of two different parts (Fig. 9.2). The outer portion, the *cortex*, consists of thousands of minute tubules called *nephrons* – these are referred to as the functioning units of the kidney. The

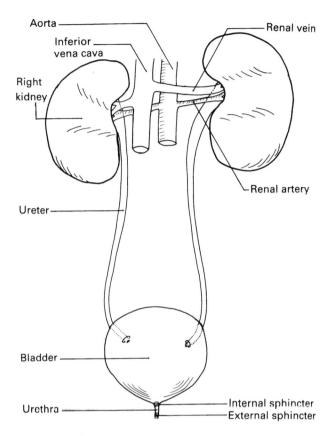

Fig. 9.1 The urinary system.

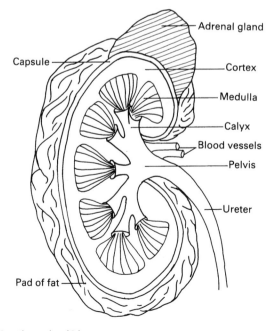

Fig. 9.2 A section through a kidney.

inner portion, the *medulla*, consists of some nephrons but also has a large collection of drainage tubules which transport the urine from the nephrons via the *calyces* to the *pelvis* of the kidney. The urine is then transported, via the ureters, to the bladder for storage. The *hilus* is the indented area of the kidney where blood vessels, lymphatic vessels and nerves enter and leave the kidney.

The blood supply to the tissue of the kidney is:

aorta → renal artery → arcuate artery → interlobular artery → afferent arteriole → glomerulus → efferent arteriole → vasa recta/peritubular capillaries → interlobular vein → arcuate vein → renal vein → inferior vena cava.

The *ureters* are two narrow tubes consisting of three layers: the innermost consisting of epithelium, the middle one of smooth muscle and the outermost of fibrous connective tissue. The ureters convey urine to the bladder by peristaltic contraction of the smooth muscle.

The *bladder* is a hollow sac made up of three layers: the innermost consisting of transitional epithelium, the middle one of smooth muscle, called the detrusor muscle, and the outer one of fibrous connective tissue. When the bladder is empty, the transitional epithelium is cuboidal and the surface of the epithelium is thrown into folds called rugae. When the bladder fills up the epithelium is flattened and stretch receptors in the wall of the bladder initiate the reflex arc (see Control of micturition). There is also an (internal) sphincter at the base of the bladder. This is composed of smooth muscle and is therefore not under voluntary control.

The *urethra* is a thin, narrow tube, some 20 cm in the male and around 3–4 cm in the female. It consists of an innermost layer of epithelium and an outer layer of submucous membrane. There is an external sphincter in the urethra, this one is made of skeletal muscle and is therefore under voluntary control. The urethra in the female is only concerned with conveying urine from the bladder to the outside of the body, whereas in the male the urethra also acts as a means of ejecting seminal fluid during sexual intercourse.

THE FUNCTIONAL UNIT OF THE KIDNEY

The functional units of the kidney, the nephrons, are twisted tubules made of specialized epithelium, the main function of which is to produce urine. Each nephron (Fig. 9.3) consists of the following parts:

■ BOX 9.1 Urinary tract infection

Infection of the urinary tract is relatively common, particularly in women, due to the shortness of the urethra and the close proximity of the anus. However, in men, urinary tract infections increase steeply from the fifth decade onwards. This is usually due to an enlargement of the prostate gland which surrounds the urethra. Infection can be confined to the bladder or can travel upwards to the kidney, resulting in pyelonephritis. In this condition severe pain is often felt in the lumber region as the inflamed, swollen kidney is being confined within the renal capsule.

Patients with an indwelling urinary catheter are at particular risk of developing a urinary tract infection. This is due to the fact that the normal defence mechanisms of the urinary tract have been bypassed, giving direct access to the body by microorganisms. A closed drainage system is used in order to cut down the risk of infection, and staff must observe stringent precautions when changing/draining bags. Staff should also note the volume, colour, turbidity and smell of the urine, and all observations should be reported accordingly.

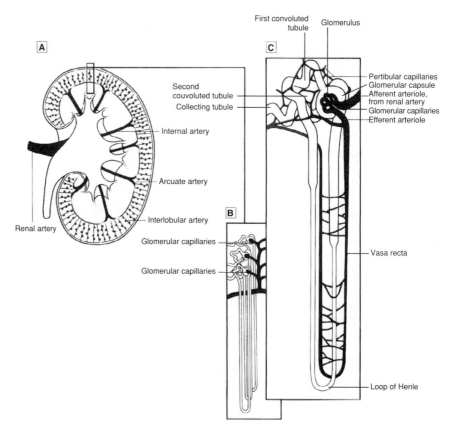

Fig. 9.3 The functional unit of the kidney: the glomerulus with associated blood supply (from Rutishauser S. Physiology and anatomy: a basis for nursing and health care. Edinburgh: Churchill Livingstone; 1994).

- a glomerular capsule
- a proximal convoluted tubule
- the loop of Henle
- distal convoluted tubule.

The distal convoluted tubules drain urine into the collecting ducts, which ultimately drain into the calyces and then into the bladder via the ureters.

Entering each *glomerular capsule* is a branch of the renal artery, referred to as the *afferent arteriole*. This vessel forms loops of capillaries, called the *glomerulus*, and finally exits from the glomerular capsule as the *efferent arteriole*. The nephron is also enmeshed by a fine capillary network called the *peritubular capillaries*, and where these capillaries enmesh the loop of Henle they are referred to as the *vasa recta*.

The glomerular capsule is composed of a single layer of epithelial cells, as is the glomerulus. This allows the passage of small solutes and water from the glomerulus to the glomerular capsule.

The *proximal convoluted tubule* consists of cuboidal epithelium which is lined with microvilli which increases the surface area for reabsorption. The *loop of Henle* is composed of two different types of epithelium and its function is concerned with water reabsorption. The *distal convoluted tubule* is composed of cuboidal epithelium and is concerned with the reabsorption of water and the secretion of ions such as H^+, K^+ and Cl^-.

THE FORMATION OF URINE

Glomerular filtration – as the efferent arteriole is narrower than the afferent arteriole the pressure within the glomerulus rises. This forces water and small solutes, such as ions, glucose and urea, from the glomerulus into the glomerular capsule. The fluid is now called *glomerular filtrate* or *tubular fluid*. Blood cells and proteins are not filtered as they are too large. Around 25% of the cardiac output goes to the kidneys, e.g. around 1250 ml/min, at rest. Of this, approximately 125 ml/min becomes tubular fluid. This is referred to as the *glomerular filtration rate*. 125 ml/min is equivalent to 180 litres/24 hours! Naturally, most of this is reabsorbed.

Selective reabsorption – takes place predominately in the proximal convoluted tubule. Nutrients such as glucose are reabsorbed from the tubular fluid and returned to the bloodstream. Most of the water is also returned, as are many ions, such as Na^+, K^+ and Cl^-.

Glucose is reabsorbed by *active transport*. This means that there has to be an upper limit, threshold or transport maximum to this process. In the case of glucose, this is 11 mmol/litre. If the glucose levels are above this, not all

---

■ **BOX 9.2 Glomerulonephritis**

Normally proteins and blood cells do not appear in the urine. However, in a condition known as glomerulonephritis blood and protein do appear. This is due to an inflammatory process which results in increased permeability of the glomerular capsule thereby permitting these large molecules to pass through. The condition can be acute or chronic.

■ **BOX 9.3 Diabetes mellitus**

In the condition known as diabetes mellitus there is an excess of glucose in the blood (hyperglycaemia) which is ultimately lost in the urine (glycosuria). The pathophysiology responsible for the condition is a lack of functioning insulin which is produced by the pancreas. Insulin is responsible for the uptake of glucose by the cells of the body, where it is used to provide energy. The body begins to utilize fats and then proteins as alternative sources of energy. Glycosuria leads to polyuria, where urine production is increased in order to excrete the excess glucose. This leads to the condition known as polydipsia which is excessive drinking, in order to prevent dehydration.

the glucose will be absorbed and glucose will appear in the urine. This is indicative of the condition known as diabetes mellitus (Box 9.3).

Approximately 80% of water and the same amount of ions are absorbed from the proximal convoluted tubule. The ions move by *passive transport* as they are moving from an area of high concentration to an area of low concentration. Water moves passively by *osmosis*. This is facilitated by the presence of the microvilli which increase surface area, therefore increasing reabsorptive capabilities.

The tubular fluid now flows into the loop of Henle, where further water reabsorption takes place. The movement of Na^+ and Cl^- at the tip of the loop creates an area of high osmotic pressure both within the tubule itself and also outwith, in the surrounding tissue fluid. The distal tubule and collecting ducts pass through this area of high osmotic pressure and water is drawn out of the tubules/ducts by osmosis and returned to the bloodstream of the vasa recta. This process is under the control of antidiuretic hormone (ADH), which is responsible for increasing the permeability of the tubules/ducts.

Specialized cells (osmoreceptors) present in the hypothalamus monitor the osmolarity (osmotic pressure) of the blood. If the osmolarity is too low, i.e. the blood is too dilute, less ADH will be released and more urine will be produced. Conversely, if the osmolarity of the blood is too high, i.e. the blood is too concentrated, then more ADH will be released and less urine will be produced.

This is the 'fine tuning' of water balance and is in line with the homeostatic needs of the body at the time in question. As much as 19 ml/min can be reabsorbed in this manner. This can perhaps be best illustrated by thinking about commonplace situations:

1. Scenario 1 – a very hot day and a lot of water is lost through sweating, therefore blood osmolarity will rise. Secretion of ADH is increased, resulting in increased permeability of the tubules/ducts. More water is reabsorbed until osmolarity returns to normal. A small volume of concentrated urine is produced.

2. Scenario 2 – large amounts of fluid drunk, resulting in a decrease in blood osmolarity. Secretion of ADH is decreased, resulting in decreased permeability of the tubules/ducts. Less water is reabsorbed until osmolarity returns to normal. A large volume of weak urine is produced.

In both instances a negative feedback mechanism exists, i.e. when the osmotic pressure returns to normal the stimuli from the osmoreceptors will cease.

Many individuals report increased urinary output after reflexology, massage or aromatherapy treatment.

Massage stimulates capillary beds and lymphatic flow, thus increasing the blood flow through the kidneys. It can also stimulate excretion of metabolic wastes, including urea and sodium chloride. Therefore there is usually increased output, with increased levels of metabolic wastes in the urine, following a massage treatment.

■ BOX 9.4 Diabetes insipidus

Diabetes insipidus is a disease caused by lack of ADH, which is normally produced by the pituitary gland. Lack of ADH results in the loss of the ability to reabsorb water from the distal convoluted tubule and the collecting ducts, resulting in a large volume of urine being produced – up to 22 litres/24 hours. Treatment is to replace ADH with a synthetic substance.

Tubular secretion – Essentially the reverse of reabsorption, where waste/ excess products are secreted from the blood into the tubular fluid. The breakdown products of drugs and hormones are removed from the blood-stream in this manner.

Excess ions are also secreted. K^+ is secreted in exchange for the reabsorption of Na^+, in order to maintain electrical balance. The amount of K^+ to be secreted is not only dependent on the amount of Na^+ to be reabsorbed but is also dependent on the amount of K^+ taken in the diet.

H^+ is also secreted in order to maintain the acid–base balance of the blood: pH 7.35–7.45 or a H^+ concentration of 36–46 nmol/litre.

THE ROLE OF THE KIDNEY IN ERYTHROPOESIS

This is stimulated by a decrease in oxygen levels within the bloodstream. Normally, red cell production is not dependent on this pathway, this is a protective measure and comes into effect if there has been a loss of blood.

A decrease in oxygen in the blood
↓
stimulates certain kidney cells
↓
to release renal erythropoetic factor
↓
which converts a plasma protein
↓
into the hormone erythropoetin
↓
which stimulates the bone marrow to increase the production of red cells.

> In the treatment of hypertension, sometimes a class of drugs called ACE inhibitors (e.g. captopril) are used. These have their effect on the renin–angiotensin–aldosterone pathway. They prevent the conversion of angiotensin I to angiotensin 2 by inactivating angiotensin converting enzyme.

THE ROLE OF THE KIDNEY IN BLOOD PRESSURE CONTROL

A drop in blood pressure or a fall in sodium
↓
stimulates the kidney to release renin
↓
which converts angiotensinogen to angiotensin 1
↓
which is then converted to angiotensin 2
↓
which stimulates the adrenal cortex to release aldosterone
↓
which reabsorbs sodium
↓
water follows by osmosis
↓
blood pressure rises.

Potassium ions are excreted as sodium ions are reabsorbed, thus maintaining electrical balance.

> In certain conditions (following general anaesthesia, after a myocardial infarction) blood pressure will drop, resulting in less blood going to the kidneys. This means that less urine will be produced and, on rare occasions, acute renal failure may develop, producing anuria. Therefore it is essential to observe urine output, sometimes on an hourly basis. Anuria is not to be confused with urinary retention, which is when urine is in the bladder but the patient cannot pass it. This could be due to a variety of factors, but sometimes a change of position and/or privacy may alleviate the problem.

CONTROL OF THE MECHANICS OF MICTURITION

When 200–300 ml of urine are present in the bladder, the stretch receptors present in the bladder wall initiate the micturition reflex. This results in contraction of muscle of the bladder and a relaxation of the internal sphincter. This is an example of a reflex arc and as such it is not under conscious control.

Almost simultaneously a message goes to the cerebral cortex and the person becomes aware of the need to micturate. If socially acceptable, the external sphincter will be voluntarily relaxed and micturition will occur. If socially unacceptable, the person will voluntarily keep the external sphincter closed. The stimuli will cease for a period of time; however, the reflex arc will return. This recurs until micturition takes place.

The conscious element is not present in the baby or toddler and micturition is purely reflex.

The examination of urine is an aid to diagnosis, not just of conditions relating to the urinary system but to systemic problems also. Every person who comes into the healthcare system should have their urine tested using the standard urinalysis 'dipstick'. Many conditions, such as diabetes mellitus and glomerulonephritis, may not have obvious presenting symptoms but can be demonstrated by testing urine.

URINE – CHARACTERISTICS AND COMPONENTS

Characteristics:

- volume, 1.5–2 litres/24 hours
- colour, yellow or amber
- turbidity, transparent when fresh
- odour, aromatic
- specific gravity, 1.001–1.035.
- pH 4.5–8.0

Components:

- water, 95%
- waste products, e.g. urea, uric acid, creatinine
- ions, e.g. Na^+, K^+, Cl^-.

URINARY SYSTEM QUESTIONS

Diagrams—Questions 434–451

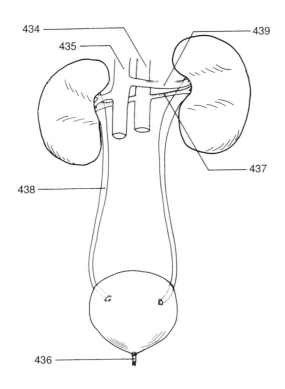

434–439. The urinary system

A. Inferior vena cava
B. Aorta
C. Renal arteries
D. Renal veins
E. Ureter
F. Urethra.

434
435
436
437
438
439

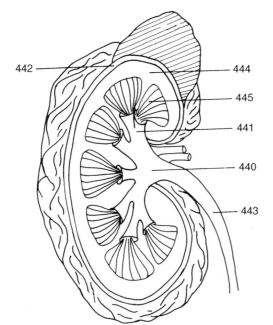

440–445. A section through the kidney

A. Cortex
B. Medulla
C. Capsule
D. Pelvis
E. Calyx
F. Ureter

440
441
442
443
444
445

446–451. A nephron

A. Glomerular
   capsule
B. Glomerulus
C. Distal
   convoluting
   tubule
D. Loop of Henle
E. Collecting tubule
F. Renal artery

446
447
448
449
450
451

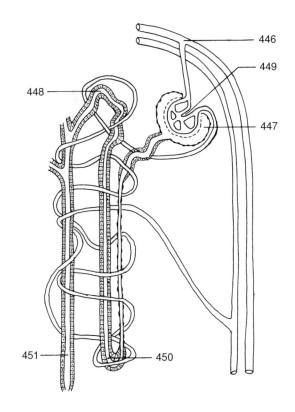

Questions 452–458 are of the multiple choice type

452. Which one of the following enters the kidney at the hilus?   452
A. Ureter
B. Renal vein
C. Renal artery
D. Lymphatic vessel.

453. Which one of the following is the part of the kidney which acts as a filter?   453
A. Loop of Henle
B. Glomerular capsule
C. The collecting tubule
D. The pelvis.

454. Which one of the following is not part of a nephron?   454
A. The calyx
B. The convoluted tubule
C. The loop of Henle
D. The collecting tubule.

**455. Which one of the following substances does not pass through the glomerular
capsule?**   455
A. Mineral salts
B. Glucose
C. Protein
D. Urea.

456. Which one of the following is correct? Normal urine: 456
A. is alkaline
B. has a specific gravity of 1050
C. contains 95% water
D. contains 2% sodium chloride.

457. The urinary bladder: 457
A. concentrates urine
B. stores urine
C. manufactures urine
D. secretes urine.

458. In glomerulonephritis the urine contains: 458
A. protein
B. bile
C. acetone
D. glucose.

Questions 459–474 are of the true/false type.   T | F

459–462. The kidney:
   459. is approximately 11 centimetres long
   460. lies behind the peritoneum
   461. lies in the iliac regions of the abdomen
   462. contains no lymphatic vessels.

463–466. The glomerulus:
   463. is cup-shaped
   464. is a collection of capillaries
   465. is a lymphatic node
   466. is part of the renal circulation.

467–470. The ureters:
   467. are continuations of the nephrons
   468. are made of voluntary muscle tissue
   469. move the urine along by peristalsis
   470. commence at the kidney pelvis.

471–474. During micturition:
   471. the abdominal wall contracts
   472. the bladder wall relaxes
   473. the internal sphincter opens
   474. the external sphincter opens by reflex action.

Questions 475–477 are of the matching items type.

475–477. From the list on the left select the statement which defines the conditions on the right.

A. The kidney is not producing urine	475. Diabetes mellitus	475
B. Absence of antidiuretic hormone	476. Diabetes insipidus	476
C. The ureter is in spasm, causing pain	477. Urinary tract infection.	477
D. Glucose appears in the urine		
E. Enlargement of the prostate gland in the male can lead to		

The nervous system

10

■ KEY POINTS

- Sensory receptors
- Neurons
- The action potential
- Synapses
- Neurotransmitters
- Brain: main parts, functional areas
- Spinal cord: reflex arc, spinal pathways

- Meninges
- Cerebrospinal fluid
- Blood supply
- Cranial/spinal nerves
- Autonomic nervous system: sympathetic nervous system, parasympathetic nervous system.

OVERVIEW

The structure and function of the nervous system is complex and not entirely understood. It is the main controlling and communicating system of the whole body and can be divided into three main parts (Fig. 10.1):

1. The *central nervous system* (CNS) consists of the brain and spinal cord. It interprets incoming information and dictates responses which are sent out from it.
2. The *peripheral nervous system* consists of nerves outside the brain and spinal cord. Sensory nerves carry information into the CNS and motor nerves carry information out of the CNS to the effector organs.
3. The *autonomic nervous system* consists of motor nerves which carry messages to effector organs that we have little control over, e.g. smooth muscles, cardiac muscle and glands.

> Bodywork therapies employ a variety of techniques that stimulate sensory receptors, such as touch, pressure, vibration and movement. Some massage techniques use reflexive mechanisms (stretch reflexes and tendon reflexes) to bring about muscular relaxation.

SENSORY RECEPTORS

These are specialized sensory nerve endings or sensory organs which register and pass on to sensory nerves the energy from many different types of stimuli. These stimuli may come from outside the body or from within it (Table 10.1).

NEURONS AND THEIR SUPPORTING CELLS

Neurons are the functional units of the nervous system and there are billions of them. They cannot divide and need constant supplies of oxygen and glucose to live. Each neuron is a nerve cell with projections of its protoplasm forming *dendrites* and one long *axon* (Fig. 10.2). The dendrites are short, branched fibres and each cell has several dendrites. The cell bodies look grey in colour, while the majority of the axons have a fatty sheath

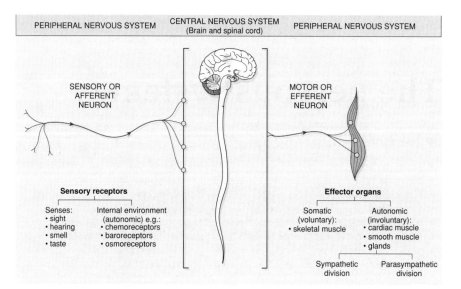

Fig. 10.1 The functional components of the nervous system (from Waugh A, Grant A. Ross and Wilson Anatomy and physiology in health and illness. 9th edn. Edinburgh: Churchill Livingstone; 2001).

Table 10.1 Examples of receptors and stimuli

Receptors	Stimuli
External sensory receptors	
Eyes	Light
Ears	Sound
Skin	Pain, temperature, pressure, touch
Internal sensory receptors	
Baroreceptors	Pressure changes
Osmoreceptors	Osmotic pressure
Chemoreceptors	Chemical changes
Thermoreceptors	Temperature

■ BOX 10.1 Multiple sclerosis

Multiple sclerosis is a condition characterized by a degeneration of the myelin sheath of the neuron. This can affect a wide variety of functions, depending upon which neurons are involved. Some common features are weak, poorly controlled muscles, disturbed sensation, e.g. pins and needles, urinary incontinence and visual disturbances. The progression of the condition is usually one of relapses and remissions.

(*myelin sheath*) which is white. This acts as an insulating material and speeds up the flow of impulses along the axon.

Neuroglia

Packed around the delicate neurons are supporting cells called *neuroglia*. There are three types of these cells: *astrocytes*, *oligodendrocytes* and *microglia*.

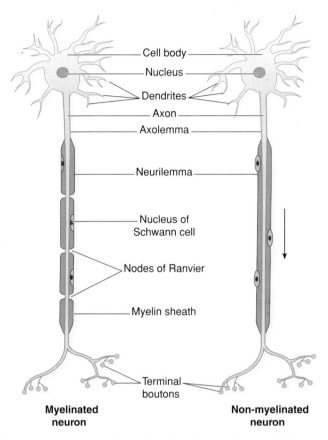

Fig. 10.2 The structure of neurons (from Waugh A, Grant A. Ross and Wilson Anatomy and physiology in health and illness. 9th edn. Edinburgh: Churchill Livingstone; 2001).

These cells are able to divide and replicate and are therefore the source of many tumours of the brain, e.g. astrocytomas.

THE ACTION POTENTIAL – NERVE IMPULSE

The sensory receptors, e.g. the eyes, are activated by a stimulus (light) and the (light) energy is transduced (changed) to form a tiny electrical charge. This electrical charge is passed along the length of the neuron. (in myelinated neurons it skips from *node of Ranvier* to node of Ranvier, i.e. quickly!). This happens due to the opening and closing of 'gates' along the nerve cell membrane, allowing negatively and positively charged ions in and out of the axon at the correct time.

The *action potential* is also continued from one neuron to the next by means of a special junction (the *synapse*) between the two.

The sensory information will be relayed in the above manner to the CNS. The brain and spinal cord will 'make sense' of the incoming information and will 'decide' if action requires to be taken (whether consciously or not). If so, a motor response will be formulated and will commence as a nerve impulse which will be transmitted, for example out of the CNS to the appropriate muscle fibre which will contract.

THE SYNAPSE

A synapse is the junction where a neuron meets another neuron. There are specialized synapses where a neuron meets muscle fibres (smooth, striped and cardiac) or glandular cells. These operate on the same principles as the neuron to neuron synapse illustrated in Figure 10.3.

The electrical impulse from the first neuron cannot 'jump' across the gap to the second neuron. Therefore a chemical (*neurotransmitter*) (*see* Fig. 10.10) is released from the axonal endings of the first neuron, fills the gap (*synaptic cleft*) and attaches to receptors on the dendrites of the second neuron. This then stimulates the second neuron and the impulse continues on its way.

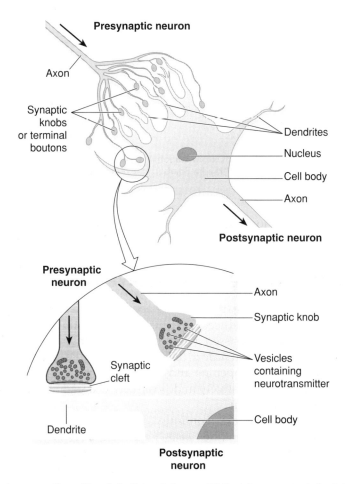

Fig. 10.3 A synapse (from Waugh A, Grant A. Ross and Wilson Anatomy and physiology in health and illness. 9th edn. Edinburgh: Churchill Livingstone; 2001).

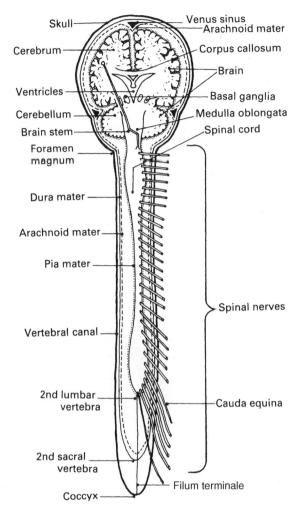

Fig. 10.4 Central nervous system.

THE CENTRAL NERVOUS SYSTEM

The central nervous system consists of the brain and spinal cord (Fig. 10.4).

The brain

The brain consists of three parts:

- the cerebrum
- the brainstem
- the cerebellum.

The cerebrum

The cerebrum is the largest part of the brain. It occupies most of the skull. It consists of two hemispheres which are joined by a bridge of white matter called the *corpus callosum*. Under the corpus callosum are the lateral *ventricles*. These are cavities in the brain which contain *cerebrospinal fluid*. The cerebrospinal fluid comes from a collection of blood capillaries in the roofs of the ventricles. This fluid circulates round the brain and spinal cord protecting and nourishing them.

The surface of the cerebrum is called the *cerebral cortex* (Fig. 10.5). It consists of billions of packed nerve cells, each with its own axon. These axons pass downwards through the lower parts of the brain into the brainstem and some continue down into the spinal cord. In the brainstem most of the axons cross each other, so that those from the left hemisphere cross to the right side of the cord and vice versa.

The cerebral cortex has a wrinkled appearance, like a walnut. The folds increase the surface area of the grey matter. It is divided into lobes by fissures. The lobes take their names from the bones beneath which they lie. Therefore each hemisphere has a frontal, parietal, temporal and occipital lobe. Fractures of the skull are named after the lobe of the brain they are overlying.

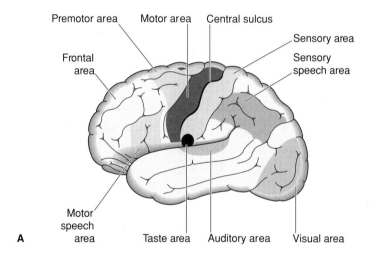

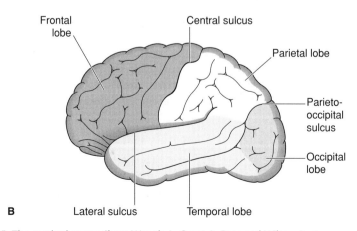

Fig. 10.5 The cerebral cortex (from Waugh A, Grant A. Ross and Wilson Anatomy and physiology in health and illness. 9th edn. Edinburgh: Churchill Livingstone; 2001).

The functions of the cerebrum are to initiate and control the movements of the skeletal muscles and to receive impulses from the sensory organs. There are groups of cells that are the emotional, thinking, reasoning and remembering centres. The grey matter of the cortex has been mapped out in great detail and certain functions attributed to the different lobes.

The areas concerned with movement are in the posterior of the frontal lobes. They are called the motor areas. The areas concerned with skin sensation are in the parietal lobes, lying alongside the motor areas but separated from them by deep fissures. The areas responsible for sight are in the occipital lobes and the hearing and smell areas are in the temporal lobes. The area for taste is in the sensory area in the parietal lobes. In the frontal lobes there are so-called silent areas which are concerned with thought, emotion, behaviour and intelligence.

The speech centre is divided into motor and sensory areas. The motor speech area is concerned with the movements required for speech, and the sensory speech area is where the spoken word is perceived. These speech centres are active in the dominant hemisphere of the brain, which is usually the left one in a right-handed person.

Dysphasia is a lack of coordination in speech, due to brain damage:

- global dysphasia – both motor and sensory speech areas affected
- expressive dysphasia – motor speech area affected
- receptive dysphasia – sensory speech area affected.

The deep layers of the cerebral cortex consist of white matter, with the exception of some groups of cells or ganglia near the base of the cerebrum. These are the *basal ganglia*, the *thalamus* and the *hypothalamus*. The basal ganglia are concerned with the coordination of muscle action. The thalamus relays sensory impulses to the brain for interpretation. The hypothalamus is associated with the pituitary gland and its hormones.

The brainstem

The brainstem connects the cerebrum to the spinal cord. It consists of three parts: the midbrain, the pons varolii and the medulla oblongata. All are vital for survival, and damage here usually results in severe consequences.

The *midbrain* is where the fibres from the two hemispheres come together. They lie in two bundles and pass under the *pons varolii*, which is a bridge of fibres connecting the two hemispheres of the cerebellum.

The *medulla oblongata* is continuous with the spinal cord and consists of white matter on the outside and grey matter on the inside. This is where most of the fibres cross over to the opposite side. This grey matter controls the heart, the blood vessels and respiration. The *cardiac centre* controls the rate and force of the heart. The *respiratory centre* controls the rate and depth of respiration. The *vaso-motor* centre controls the muscular walls of the small blood vessels, causing vasoconstriction or vasodilation to occur.

There are also *reflex centres* in the medulla oblongata. These initiate coughing, sneezing and vomiting when something is irritating the respiratory tract or the stomach.

The aim of carrying out neurological observations is to detect, at an early stage, deterioration or improvement in conscious level. The Glasgow Coma Scale is a universally accepted tool which is used as an objective measurement of this. Three types of behaviour are assessed: eye-opening, verbal response and motor response. Observations of vital signs, temperature, pulse, blood pressure and respirations are also carried out. Any change, however slight, must be reported and acted upon to avoid serious consequences.

■ **BOX 10.2 Stroke**

'Stroke' is a term used to describe a cerebrovascular accident which results from an interruption of blood flow to the brain followed by death of brain tissue. It is commonly due to the blockage of an artery by a thrombus or atheromatous plaque. The severity of the stroke and the resulting signs and symptoms depend upon the location of the accident and how large an area of brain is supplied by the affected vessel. Frequent signs and symptoms are paralysis of one side of the body, sensory and speech disturbances.

The cerebellum

The cerebellum is the hindbrain. It is situated at the back, beneath the occipital lobe of the cerebrum. Like the cerebrum, it has grey matter on the outside and white matter inside. It consists of two hemispheres joined by a bridge of fibres called the *vermis*.

The cerebellum is connected to the cerebrum, the brainstem and the spinal cord. Its functions are coordination of muscle movement, balance and maintaining the tone of the muscles so that they are ready for immediate action. Watch a child learning to ride a bicycle and think of the functions of the cerebellum.

The blood supply to the brain

The carotid arteries and the vertebral arteries supply blood to the brain. These arteries branch and join up again, forming a circle of arteries at the base of the brain called the *circle of Willis*. From here smaller *cerebral* arteries branch off to supply each region of the brain.

Blood returns from the brain to the superior vena cava by the *jugular veins*. The venous blood collects in channels called the *venous sinuses* which lie between the two layers of the dura mater (see p. 218). From these venous sinuses the blood drains into the jugular veins.

The spinal cord

The spinal cord is a continuation of the brainstem. It lies in the vertebral canal, extending from the foramen magnum to between the first and second lumbar vertebrae. It is cylindrical, approximately 45 cm long and about the same thickness as the little finger.

The spinal cord consists of grey matter on the inside and white matter on the outside. The grey matter continues through the whole length of the spinal cord, rather like the lettering in a stick of rock. In section it is roughly the shape of the letter 'H'. There is a tiny central canal which is continuous with the ventricles of the brain and contains cerebrospinal fluid.

From the cells in the grey matter come the fibres that form the spinal or peripheral nerves. The anterior horns of the grey matter (see Fig. 10.6) contain the cells of the motor neurons which supply the muscles and glands. The posterior horns contain the cells of the sensory neurons which supply the skin and other sensory organs. The beginnings of the axons from these cells are called the motor and sensory roots. They form the roots of the spinal nerves. The roots come together just as they leave the vertebral canal, where they are bound in a common sheath to form a nerve. Injury to a nerve will, therefore, cause loss of sensation as well as of movement.

The white matter of the spinal cord consists of nerve fibres or axons lying in anterior, posterior and lateral columns. These are the fibres which form the sensory and motor pathways to and from the brain.

The sensory and motor pathways

Consider what happens when you touch something unpleasant and decide to withdraw your hand. The sensory nerve endings in the skin are stimulated by the object. An impulse passes up the peripheral nerve into the posterior horns of the spinal cord. From here the impulse is transmitted to the white matter where it travels up another sensory neuron to the thalamus where the sensation is felt, but only crudely. From the thalamus, the sensation is relayed by another neuron to the sensory area of the cortex of the brain where the fine sensation is interpreted. There are, therefore, three different lots of sensory neurons involved before you can feel the exact temperature, shape and texture of an object.

To withdraw the hand, impulses pass down from the brain through two groups of motor neurons. The *upper motor neurons* have their cells in the cerebral cortex and their axons in the brain, brainstem and spinal cord. The impulses pass from the brain down the cord to the level at which the spinal nerve leaves. If the nerve is supplying muscle of the lower limbs, the axon will continue to the end of the cord. When it is the upper limb you wish to move, the axons will stop in the neck. The impulses will then be transmitted to the cells in the anterior horn of the grey matter and a second or *lower motor neuron* will convey the impulse to the muscles by the peripheral nerves. The muscles will contract and produce the required movement.

Reflex arc

There are occasions when the movements of voluntary muscles are not controlled by the brain. In the grey matter of the spinal cord, between the cells of the anterior and posterior horns, are small connector neurons which will transmit an impulse straight from the skin to muscles (see Fig. 10.6). This is called reflex arc and it occurs if you touch something which is dangerous. You will have withdrawn your hand before you are aware of unacceptable heat or pain. However, the information is received by the brain milliseconds later.

The meninges

The meninges are protective coverings for the brain and the spinal cord. There are three membranes. The outer one lines the skull and vertebral canal as far as the second sacral vertebra and is called the *dura mater*. The other two lie between the dura mater and the brain and spinal cord. They are the *arachnoid mater* and the *pia mater*.

The dura mater

The dura mater consists of two layers of tough fibrous tissue. The two layers are close together except where the inner layer dips down between

Epidural analgesia is the administration of analgesics and anti-inflammatory drugs into the epidural space. This space lies outside the dura mater and is transversed by the spinal nerves. Some indications for its use include provision of analgesia during labour, as an alternative to general anaesthesia and to provide adequate postoperative analgesia.

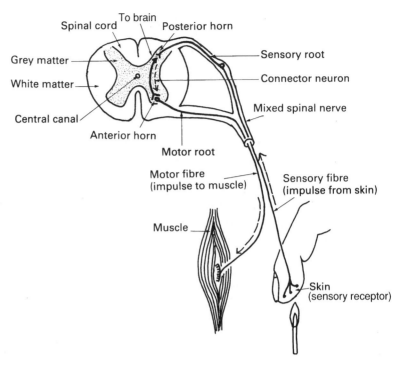

Fig. 10.6 Diagrammatic section of spinal cord to show a reflex arc.

■ BOX 10.3 Meningitis

The meninges can be infected by a variety of blood-borne microorganisms. They cause inflammation of the pia mater and arachnoid mater (meningitis). Symptoms can include headaches, vomiting and reflex spasm of spinal muscles. Complications of the infection may occur, such as a rash, high temperature and septicaemia, which can lead to severe shock and even death.

---

the hemispheres of the cerebrum and between the cerebellum and the cerebrum (see Fig. 10.4). At these points the dura mater forms the venous sinuses, the channels into which the venous blood drains (see p. 216).

The arachnoid mater

The arachnoid mater, so called because it resembles a spider's web, is a fine covering of serous membrane which lies under the dura mater. It is separated from the dura mater by a potential space called the subdural space. It covers the brain and spinal cord and extends down to the second sacral vertebra.

The pia mater

The pia mater is a fine membrane, consisting of minute blood vessels held together by areolar tissue. The pia mater covers the brain and dips down between the convolutions and fissures on the brain surface. It covers the spinal cord and continues down as a thread like structure from the end of the cord to fuse with the sacrum. This thread is called the *filum terminale*, and it helps to anchor the cord, preventing unnecessary movement.

■ BOX 10.4 Hydrocephalus

Excess cerebrospinal fluid is known as hydrocephalus. It may be due to overproduction of cerebrospinal fluid, reduction in its reabsorption or obstruction to its flow. A simple device known as a shunt may be inserted into one of the ventricles to divert the excess. If left untreated for any length of time, it can cause brain damage.

Cerebrospinal fluid

Between the arachnoid mater and the pia mater is a space called the *subarachnoid space*. This space contains *cerebrospinal fluid*, a clear watery fluid containing mineral salts and traces of protein and glucose. The fluid is secreted into the *ventricles* of the brain from capillaries (called choroid plexuses) in the roof of each ventricle. There are four ventricles. The two lateral ventricles have already been discussed. The third ventricle lies below them and the fourth lies between the cerebellum and the pons varolii.

Cerebrospinal fluid circulates from the ventricles round the brain and spinal cord, acting as a water cushion or shock absorber. It protects these delicate structures from contact injury with the hard skull and the walls of the vertebral canal. It is reabsorbed at the same rate it is made through special channels in the arachnoid mater and is then returned to the venous blood supply.

The subarachnoid space below the end of the cord contains cerebrospinal fluid and the roots of the nerves which supply the lower limbs. This collection of roots resembles the coarse hair of a horse's tail, which is why it is called the *cauda equina*.

THE PERIPHERAL NERVOUS SYSTEM

The peripheral nervous system consists of the nerves that leave the brainstem and spinal cord. There are 12 pairs of *cranial nerves* mainly supplying the structures above the neck. The trunk and limbs are supplied by 31 pairs of *spinal nerves*.

The cranial nerves

There are 12 pairs of cranial nerves leaving the brainstem. Four pairs of these nerves supply the sensory organs in the skull.

- the *olfactory* nerve is the nerve of smell
- the *glossopharangeal* nerve is the nerve of taste
- the *vestibulocochlear* nerve is the nerve of hearing and balance
- the *optic* nerve is the nerve of sight.

Lumbar puncture is the withdrawal of cerebrospinal fluid from the lumbar subarachnoid space via a hollow spinal needle. It is usually carried out between the second and third lumbar vertebrae, i.e. below the level of the actual spinal cord. It may be done to diagnose illness, for radiological purposes or to introduce drugs into the cerebrospinal fluid. Careful positioning to ensure maximum widening of the intervertebral spaces must be undertaken as this gives easier access to the subarachnoid space. This may be lying, with head flexed and knees drawn up, or, more rarely, sitting. Support, encouragement and careful observation will be required throughout the procedure.

Three pairs of cranial nerves supply the muscles that move the eyeballs, an important part of facial expression. Facial expression also includes movement of the facial muscles which are supplied by the facial nerve. The trigeminal nerve supplies the skin of the face and the muscles of mastication. Other cranial nerves supply the muscles that move the head and the tongue.

The *vagus* nerve is the only cranial nerve which passes into the trunk. This is a sensory and motor nerve which supplies the organs of the thorax and abdomen. It is part of the autonomic nervous system.

The spinal nerves

The spinal nerves pass out of the vertebral canal, one pair emerging below each vertebra and one pair emerging between the cranium and the first cervical vertebra. This gives:

- eight pairs of cervical nerves
- 12 pairs of thoracic nerves
- five pairs of lumbar nerves
- five pairs of sacral nerves
- one pair of coccygeal nerves.

The lumbar, sacral and coccygeal nerves pass straight down from the end of the spinal cord to reach their respective exit foramina. The roots of these nerves form the cauda equina (see Fig. 10.4).

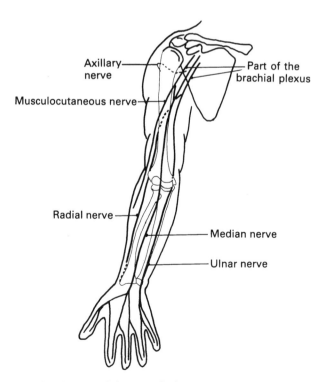

Fig. 10.7 The peripheral nerves of the upper limb.

Each nerve contains motor and sensory fibres. They come from the cells in the anterior and posterior horns of the grey matter of the spinal cord. As these fibres leave the cord they form the motor and sensory roots. The roots come together as they leave the vertebral canal to form the spinal nerves. A spinal nerve consists of bundles of nerve fibres wrapped up in connective tissue for protection. Before the nerves reach the limbs they form networks, rather like railway junctions. Each of these networks is called a *plexus*.

The nerves from the *cervical plexus* supply the skin and the muscles of the neck.

The nerves from the *brachial plexus* supply the upper limbs (Fig. 10.7). The brachial plexus lies in the axilla and has five branches. The *radial* nerve, which supplies the extensor muscles of the wrist and fingers, has already been mentioned because it can be damaged so easily by careless handling of an unconscious patient (see Box 2.10). The *median* nerve supplies the flexor muscles of the wrist and fingers and thumb. The *ulnar* nerve supplies the muscles of the hand and the *axillary* nerve supplies the muscles that move the shoulders. The *musculocutaneous* nerve supplies the biceps muscle which flexes the elbow. These nerves also supply some part of the skin of the upper limbs.

The thoracic nerves do not form a plexus but pass round the chest wall protected by the ribs. They supply the muscles and skin of the thorax and abdomen.

The *lumbar plexus* has two main branches. The *femoral* nerve supplies the quadriceps muscle which extends the knee, and the *obturator* nerve supplies the adductor muscles of the hip.

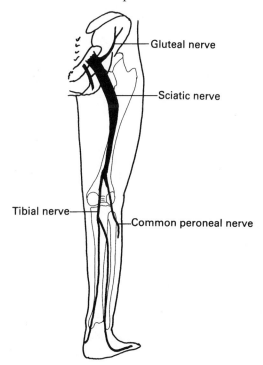

Gluteal nerve

Sciatic nerve

Tibial nerve

Common peroneal nerve

Fig. 10.8 The peripheral nerves of the lower limb.

The sciatic nerve is the largest nerve in the body and is the nerve that can be damaged by an incorrectly given intramuscular injection into the buttock.

The *sacral plexus* has one large branch, the *sciatic* nerve, and some smaller branches, the *gluteal* nerves (Fig. 10.8). The gluteal nerves supply the muscles of the hip. The sciatic nerve supplies the hamstring muscles which flex the knee and all the muscles below the knee which act on the ankle joint and toes. The *common peroneal nerve* is a branch of the sciatic nerve. Injury to this nerve at the point where it winds round the lateral aspect of the knee may be the cause of dropped foot. Pressure on this nerve gives you 'pins and needles' if you sit too long with your knees crossed. The skin of the lower limbs and pelvis is supplied by nerves from the lumbar and sacral plexuses.

THE AUTONOMIC NERVOUS SYSTEM

The autonomic nervous system (ANS) is the part of the nervous system which supplies smooth muscle, cardiac muscle and the glands of the body. It controls the movements of the internal organs and the secretions of the glands. We have little or no control over this part of the nervous system. Almost all of the tissues supplied by the ANS have two sets of nerves supplying them. One from the sympathetic nervous system and one from the parasympathetic nervous system. One of these systems acts to increase the activity of the tissue and the other acts to decrease the activity. Therefore the activity of the muscle or gland is normally kept in balance. The autonomic nerve cells are situated in the brainstem and

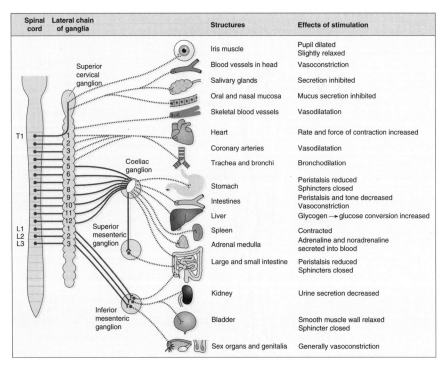

Spinal cord	Lateral chain of ganglia	Structures	Effects of stimulation
	Superior cervical ganglion	Iris muscle	Pupil dilated Slightly relaxed
		Blood vessels in head	Vasoconstriction
		Salivary glands	Secretion inhibited
		Oral and nasal mucosa	Mucus secretion inhibited
		Skeletal blood vessels	Vasodilatation
T1 1 2 3 4 5 6 7 8 9 10 11 12	Coeliac ganglion	Heart	Rate and force of contraction increased
		Coronary arteries	Vasodilatation
		Trachea and bronchi	Bronchodilation
		Stomach	Peristalsis reduced Sphincters closed
		Intestines	Peristalsis and tone decreased Vasoconstriction
		Liver	Glycogen → glucose conversion increased
L1 L2 L3 1 2 3	Superior mesenteric ganglion	Spleen	Contracted
		Adrenal medulla	Adrenaline and noradrenaline secreted into blood
		Large and small intestine	Peristalsis reduced Sphincters closed
		Kidney	Urine secretion decreased
	Inferior mesenteric ganglion	Bladder	Smooth muscle wall relaxed Sphincter closed
		Sex organs and genitalia	Generally vasoconstriction

Fig. 10.9 The sympathetic nervous system (from Waugh A, Grant A. Ross and Wilson Anatomy and physiology in health and illness. 9th edn. Edinburgh: Churchill Livingstone; 2001).

spinal cord. The axons leave the brainstem and spinal cord with the peripheral nerves.

The sympathetic nervous system

Commonly known as the 'fight or flight' system. Activity of this system increases when a person is under stress (whether pleasurable or frightening). This activity is aimed at getting the person out of the situation or in helping them cope with it.

Before being distributed to the various organs, the fibres of the sympathetic nervous system enter a chain of ganglia which lie on either side of the vertebral column (Fig. 10.9). This ensures that the first neuron, carrying an impulse, reaching the chain will synapse with not only the second neuron, which will carry the impulse to the organ, but also with neurons running up and down the chain. These will, in turn, synapse with all the second neurons in the system and therefore all of the organs will activate at once. This is essential in cases of extreme danger.

From the CNS to the actual effector organ there are two synapses, one between neuron one and neuron two, and one between neuron two and the effector organ. Therefore two neurotransmitters are required to transmit the impulse and actually operate the organ (Fig. 10.10).

> Bodywork treatments initially stimulate the sympathetic nervous system and, as a consequence, homeostatic mechanisms elicit parasympathetic responses. Therefore massage can be either stimulating or sedative, depending on the type of manipulations used.

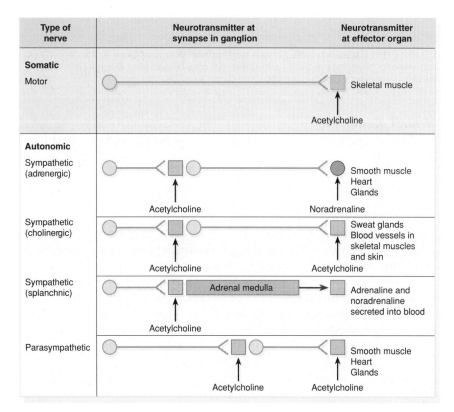

Fig. 10.10 Neurotransmitters at synapses in the peripheral nervous system (from Waugh A, Grant A. Ross and Wilson Anatomy and physiology in health and illness. 9th edn. Edinburgh: Churchill Livingstone; 2001).

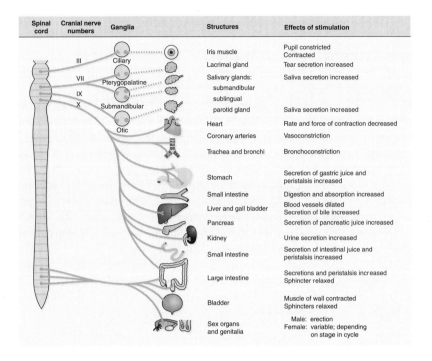

Fig. 10.11 The parasympathetic nervous system (from Waugh A, Grant A. Ross and Wilson Anatomy and physiology in health and illness. 9th edn. Edinburgh: Churchill Livingstone; 2001).

> The *chakras* (energy centres) of ayurvedic medicine and some of the *acupuncture* points (the *back-shu* points) of traditional Chinese medicine are located at the ganglia of the parasympathetic nervous system. Many complementary therapists use techniques such as acupressure to stimulate these ganglia on either side of the spine.

Adrenal gland

The sympathetic nervous system also supplies the adrenal glands situated on top of each of the kidneys. These glands (amongst other things) produce adrenaline and noradrenaline which circulate in the bloodstream and augment all the activities of the sympathetic nervous system.

The parasympathetic nervous system

The parasympathetic nervous system is more straightforward than the sympathetic nervous system as it has no chain of ganglia and no augmenting gland. Its influence tends to dominate when you are rested and relaxed. As can be seen from Figure 10.11, it is mainly involved in digestion and maintenance functions of the body. There are still two neurons from the CNS to the effector organs, therefore this system also has two synapses and two neurotransmitters (see Fig. 10.10).

NERVOUS SYSTEM QUESTIONS

Diagrams—Questions 478–481

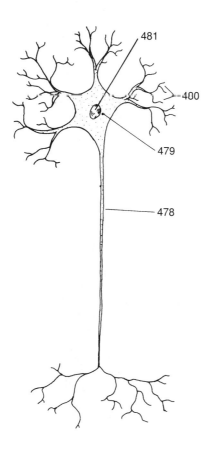

478–481. A neuron

A. Dendrite
B. Axon
C. Nucleus
D. Cell

478
479
480
481

482–493. Central nervous system

A. Cerebrum
B. Cerebellum
C. Ventricles
D. Medulla
   oblongata
E. Spinal cord
F. Cauda equina
G. Filum terminale
H. Pia mater
I. Dura mater
J. Foramen
   magnum
K. A thoracic nerve
L. A lumbar nerve

482
483
484
485
486
487
488
489
490
491
492
493

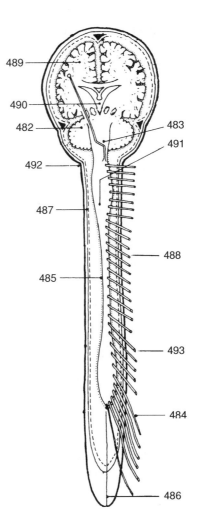

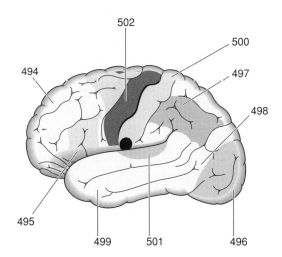

494–502. The cerebral cortex

A. Frontal lobe
B. Parietal lobe
C. Temporal lobe
D. Occipital lobe
E. Motor area
F. Sensory area
G. Visual area
H. Auditory area
I. Motor speech area

494
495
496
497
498
499
500
501
502

503–509. Section through spinal cord

A. Posterior root
B. Anterior root
C. Posterior horn
D. Connector neuron
E. Spinal nerve
F. Motor nerve ending
G. Central canal

| 503 |
| 504 |
| 505 |
| 506 |
| 507 |
| 508 |
| 509 |

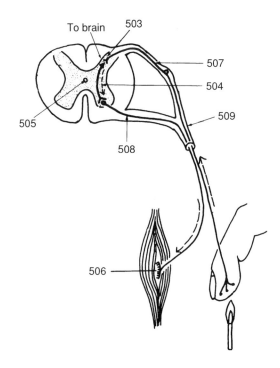

510–513. Peripheral nerves

A. Brachial plexus
B. Radial nerve
C. Median nerve
D. Ulnar nerve

| 510 |
| 511 |
| 512 |
| 513 |

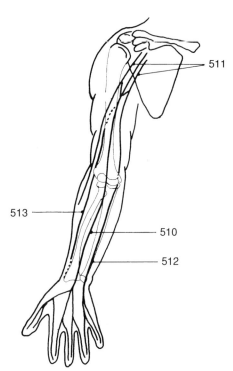

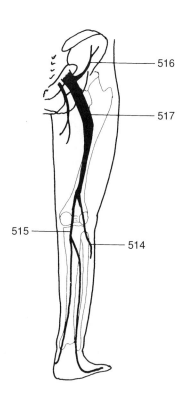

514–517.

A. Sciatic nerve
B. Common
    peroneal nerve
C. Gluteal nerve
D. Tibial nerve

514
515
516
517

Questions 518–522 are of the multiple choice type

518. The unit of the nervous system is a: 518
  A. nephron
  B. neutron
  C. neuron
  D. nerve.

519. Which one of the following is the fatty covering of an axon?   519
  A. Neuroglia
  B. Neurilemma
  C. Myelin sheath
  D. Adipose tissue.

520. The venous sinuses of the brain lie between the: 520
  A. dura mater and the skull
  B. inner and outer layers of the dura mater
  C. arachnoid mater and the pia mater
  D. dura mater and the arachnoid mater.

521. Which one of the following is a function of the sympathetic nervous system?
Constriction of the: 521
  A. bronchioles
  B. coronary artery
  C. skin arterioles
  D. pupils.

522. Which one of the following is a function of the parasympathetic nervous system?   522
  A. The heart beat is increased
  B. The blood pressure rises
  C. There is an increase in the flow of saliva
  D. The secretion of gastric juice decreases.

Questions 523–554 are of the true/false type   T | F

523–526. The central nervous system controls:
523. growth
524. the movement of the skeleton
525. the flow of gastric juice
526. peristalsis.

527–530. From which of the following arteries does the brain receive its blood supply?
527. Carotid
528. Facial
529. Subclavian
530. Vertebral.

531–534. The cerebrum:
531. has two hemispheres
532. is composed entirely of grey matter
533. is divided into six lobes
534. is protected by cerebrospinal fluid.

535–538. The spinal cord:
535. is about 45 cm long
536. extends to the end of the vertebral canal
537. contains a central canal
538. has grey matter on the outside.

539–542. The cranial nerves:
539. lie entirely within the skull
540. number 12 pairs
541. have their roots in the spinal cord
542. are all motor nerves.

543–546. The spinal nerves:
543. number 32 pairs
544. are all mixed nerves
545. form plexuses
546. supply the internal organs.

547–550. The brachial plexus:
547. lies in the axilla
548. has two branches
549. supplies the chest wall
550. supplies the upper limb.

551–554. The branches of the sacral plexus form the:
551. femoral nerve
552. gluteal nerve
553. obturator nerve
554. sciatic nerve.

Questions 555–572 are of the matching items type.

555–557. From the list on the left select the function associated with each lobe of the cerebrum listed on the right.

A. Hearing	555. Frontal	555
B. Sight	556. Parietal	556
C. Movement	557. Occipital.	557
D. Touch		
E. Smell		

558–560. From the list on the left select the statement which relates to each part of the brainstem listed on the right.

A. Connects the cerebellar hemispheres	558. Midbrain	558
B. Contains the hypothalamus	559. Pons varolii	559
C. Is where the fibres cross	560. Medulla oblongata.	560
D. Contains motor speech area		
E. Is the uppermost part of the brainstem		

561–563. From the list on the left select the statement which describes each of the structures listed on the right.

A. Lines the skull and vertebral canal	561. Arachnoid mater	561
B. Consists of serous membrane	562. Pia mater	562
C. Secretes cerebrospinal fluid	563. Dura mater.	563
D. Forms the filum terminale		
E. Forms the cauda equina		

564–566. From the list on the left select the contents of the parts of the spinal cord listed on the right.

A. Motor fibres only	564. Anterior horns	564
B. Motor cells	565. Posterior horns	565
C. Sensory and motor fibres	566. Columns of white matter.	566
D. Sensory cells		
E. Sympathetic nerves		

567–569. From the list on the left select the statement which describes the action of each structure listed on the right.

A. Connects the muscles to the brain	567. Motor pathway	567
B. Connects the eyes to the brain	568. Sensory pathway	568
C. Connects two different neurons	569. Connector neuron.	569
D. Connects the brain to the muscles		
E. Connects the skin to the brain		

570–572. From the list on the left select the part supplied by the nerves listed on the right.

A. Extensors of the wrist	570. Axillary	570
B. Shoulder muscles	571. Median	571
C. Muscles of the hand	572. Radial.	572
D. Thumb		
E. Flexors of the elbow		

The special senses

11

■ KEY POINTS

- The eye and vision
- The ear, hearing and balance
- The nose and smell
- The tongue and taste (see Ch. 7)
- The skin and touch (see Ch. 8).

THE EYE AND VISION

The eye is the organ of sight. It is concerned with receiving rays of light reflected back from objects in the environment. The nerve endings in the eyeball are stimulated by the light. The optic nerve (second cranial nerve) carries these impulses back to the occipital lobes of the cerebral cortex where they are interpreted.

The eyeball

The eyeballs are almost spherical in shape. They lie in the cone-shaped orbits within the skull, protected by the eyelids to the front, a pad of fat at the back and the dense bony orbit.

Each eyeball is attached to the orbit by six small muscles which move the eyes. These extrinsic muscles act together so that both eyeballs move simultaneously in the same direction. If there is a weakness of one muscle, the eye will squint. This is called a *strabismus*.

The eyeball has three coats or layers and the centre is a chamber filled with a jelly-like substance (the vitreous body or humour). The

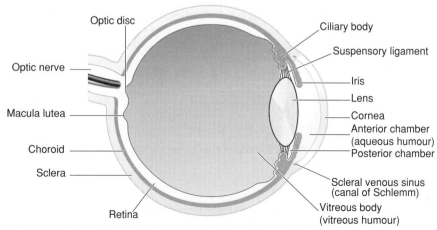

Fig. 11.1 Section of the eye (from Waugh A, Grant A. Ross and Wilson Anatomy and physiology in health and illness. 9th edn. Edinburgh: Churchill Livingstone; 2001).

coats, from the outer coat inwards, are the *sclera*, the *choroid* and the *retina* (Fig. 11.1).

The sclera and cornea

The outer coat of the eyeball is tough and fibrous and is protective in function. It maintains the shape of the eyeball and provides attachment for the extrinsic muscles. It consists of two parts: the larger posterior part is opaque, it forms the white part of the eye and is called the sclera. The anterior part is transparent and is called the *cornea*. The cornea allows the rays of light to pass into the eyeball. It is very sensitive and the slightest spot of dust touching it will cause the eyelid to come down like a shutter. This blinking action helps to keep the eyeball clean and aids in its protection.

The choroid

The choroid is the coloured part of the eyeball. It lines the posterior part of the inner surface of the sclera. It is rich in blood vessels and is dark brown in colour. This dark colour prevents the rays of light which have entered the eye from being reflected out again.

The choroid lines the sclera and also forms the *iris*. The iris lies between the cornea and the *lens*. It is like a circular curtain with a hole in the middle called the *pupil*. Behind the iris is a circular muscle called the *ciliary body*. This muscle has *suspensory ligaments* attached to it which hold the lens in place. The ciliary body, by contracting and relaxing, can alter the shape of the lens. It also secretes a watery fluid called *aqueous humour* which is contained in the *anterior* and *posterior chambers* of the eyeball. This fluid passes back into the circulatory system via a small canal, called the canal of *Schlemm*, which is situated in the angle between the iris and cornea. The anterior chamber is the space between the cornea and iris. The posterior chamber lies between the iris and the lens.

■ BOX 11.1 Glaucoma

Glaucoma is a disease characterized by raised pressure within the eye, usually caused by impaired drainage of aqueous humour into the canal of Schlemm. This raised pressure causes damage to the neurons of the optic disc, leading to eventual blindness. It may be treated with drugs and/or surgery.

The lens

The lens is a colourless, transparent, biconvex, elastic structure enclosed in a transparent capsule. It lies between the aqueous humour and the *vitreous*

■ BOX 11.2 Cataract

A cataract is an opacity of the lens of the eye which may be degenerative or congenital in origin. The visual impairment can vary in extent, but can lead to eventual blindness which is treated by surgical removal of the lens.

humour, which is the jelly-like substance contained in the cavity of the eyeball.

The retina

The retina is the light-sensitive inner coat of the eyeball. It consists of a pigmented layer of tissue which attaches it to the choroid. In front of this tissue is a network of nerve cells and fibres and a layer of light-sensitive cells called *rods* and *cones*. There are millions of rods and cones in each eyeball. Most of the cones are clustered together at the back of the retina, where they form a very sensitive area called the *macula lutea*. When you look directly at something, the rays of light from that object are focused on the centre of the macula and the object appears clearer than its surroundings.

The cones are sensitive to bright light and colour. The rods are sensitive to dim light and movement, and they contain a substance called *visual purple*. Visual purple prevents night blindness and requires the intake of vitamin A to maintain its effectiveness.

Beside the macula is the *blind spot*. This is where the optic nerve leaves the eye and there are no nerve cells. We do not see it as a blind spot because we see with both eyes at once. One eye compensates for the blind spot of the other. The optic nerve from each eyeball passes back into the skull and they come together at the base of the brain – the *optic chiasma*. Some of the nerve fibres cross at this point so that the nerves that eventually reach the right and left occipital cortex contain fibres from both eyes.

Seeing with both eyes (binocular vision) produces three-dimensional vision. You can judge distance, height and depth much better. It is called *stereoscopic vision*.

Vision

When rays of light pass from one substance to another of different density, they bend. If you stand a stick in a pool of water, the stick will look as if it bends as it enters the water. This bending of light rays is called refraction and is the reason we can see. Light rays entering the eyeball pass through the cornea, the aqueous humour, the lens and the vitreous humour. These substances all bend the rays so that they become focused on the retina (Fig. 11.2).

The lens is adjustable, allowing the rays of light to be bent as necessary. If you are looking at a close object, the rays must be bent through a greater angle than if you are looking at a distant object. For reading, therefore, the lens must be thicker. The ciliary muscle contracts and the lens becomes more convex. Lifting the head and looking into the distance relaxes the muscle and keeps the eyes from getting too tired.

■ BOX 11.3 Myopia

Myopia or nearsightedness occurs when the eyeball is too long and the image is formed in front of the retina. Correction is achieved by using a concave lens which allows objects to be seen in focus.

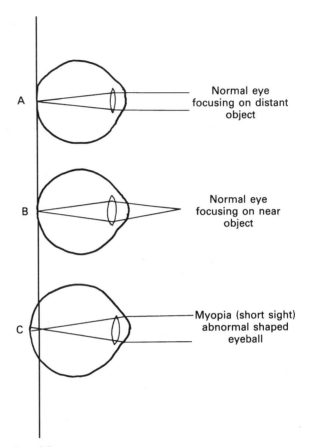

A — Normal eye focusing on distant object

B — Normal eye focusing on near object

C — Myopia (short sight) abnormal shaped eyeball

Fig. 11.2 Focusing of the eye.

Focusing the eyes is called accommodation. Accommodation depends on the shape of the lens, movement of the eyes and the size of the pupil. The two types of muscle fibres of the iris are circular and radiating. When the radiating muscle fibres contract under the influence of the sympathetic nervous system, the pupils dilate and more light enters the eyes. When the circular fibres contract, the pupil constricts and less light enters. The circular muscle fibres are influenced by the parasympathetic nervous system.

The protective structures of the eye

The eye is a very delicate organ and it is protected by several structures. The fact that it lies in a bony cavity, which is softened at the back by a pad of fat, prevents direct injury. The other structures which give protection are the eyelids, the eyebrows and the tear glands (Fig. 11.3). The eyelids are like shutters. They are muscular, are covered with skin and can be opened and closed at will. The edges of the eyelids are covered in hairs – the eyelashes – which help to keep out dust, foreign bodies and too much light. If an object approaches the eye suddenly, the lids automatically close and the eyelashes help to sweep the object away.

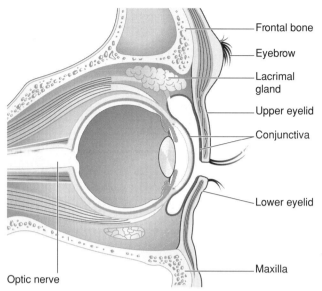

Labels on figure:
Frontal bone
Eyebrow
Lacrimal gland
Upper eyelid
Conjunctiva
Lower eyelid
Maxilla
Optic nerve

Fig. 11.3 Section of the eye and its accessory structures (from Waugh A, Grant A. Ross and Wilson Anatomy and physiology in health and illness. 9th edn. Edinburgh: Churchill Livingstone; 2001).

Covering the front of the eyeball and lining the eyelids is a thin layer of transparent mucous membrane called the *conjunctiva*. Any speck of dust which has not been swept away by the eyelashes will stick to the conjunctiva and can be removed without damaging the eye itself.

The eyebrows help cut down the amount of light entering the eye. This is why we frown when the light is too bright. They also help prevent sweat from running down into the eyes.

A foreign body in the eye makes the eye 'weep', not always because it is so painful but more as a reflex attempt to wash away the irritating object. Situated above each eye is a small gland called the *lacrimal gland* (Fig. 11.4). This gland secretes tears. Tears are a salty fluid which flow over the front of the eye, continually washing it. Tears contain a substance called *lysozyme*, which helps to kill off any microorganisms. Normally the tears flow towards the nasal side of the eye where they enter the *lacrimal sac* before passing down the *lacrimal duct* and being evaporated in the nose. It is only when the eye is injured or when we are emotionally upset that we are aware of the tears. The lacrimal gland then produces additional fluid which overflows and runs down the cheeks.

THE EAR, HEARING AND BALANCE

The ear is the organ of hearing and of balance, although actual interpretation of sound is carried out by the brain. The ear is constructed in such a way that the sound waves passing through the atmosphere are caught up by the ears and the resulting electrical impulses are transmitted to the hearing centre in the temporal lobe of the cerebral cortex. The ear consists of three main parts: the outer, middle and inner ear (Fig. 11.5).

Eye drops are usually instilled into the lower fornix of the eye. The hands should be thoroughly washed prior to undertaking this procedure and care should be taken to use the correctly prescribed drops for the correct eye. The dropper should be held as close to the eye as is possible without touching either the lids or the cornea. Ideally single-dose containers should be used to prevent infection.

When cleaning eyes, hands must be thoroughly washed prior to undertaking the procedure. The cleanest or non-infected eye is always dealt with first. Swabbing is carried out on a closed eye first before asking the patient to look up (for lower lid) and look down (for upper lid) to enable cleaning of the lid margins. The eye is cleaned from the nasal corner outwards as this will reduce the risk of debris being swept into the lacrimal punctum or, accidently, into the other eye.

The best position for installing ear drops is lying on one side with the ear to be treated uppermost. Drops may be prescribed for individual ears. Warming of the drops is preferable, if possible. Straighten the external acoustic canal by gently pulling the cartilaginous part of the auricle backwards and upwards, instill the drops as prescribed, and request that the position is maintained for 1–2 minutes to prevent the drops running back out again.

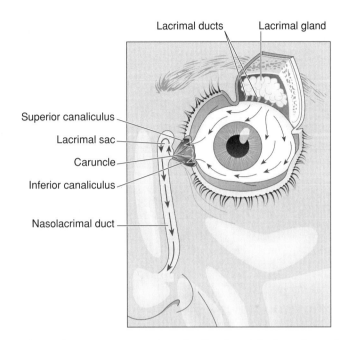

Fig. 11.4 The lacrimal apparatus. Arrows show the direction of the flow of tears (from Waugh A, Grant A. Ross and Wilson Anatomy and physiology in health and illness. 9th edn. Edinburgh: Churchill Livingstone; 2001).

The outer ear

The visible part of the ear is the *auricle*. The auricle is a collecting trumpet for the sound waves. It is composed of elastic fibrocartilage covered with skin.

The more important parts of the ear lie within the temporal bone. From the auricle a curved canal, the *external acoustic meatus*, leads towards the *eardrum*. This canal is partly cartilage and partly bone. It is lined with skin from which hairs grow, and it contains small glands which secrete wax. The curve in the canal, the hairs and the wax are all protective in function and help to prevent foreign bodies from reaching the eardrum. The external acoustic meatus ends at the *tympanic membrane* which is the eardrum. The tympanic membrane is composed of fibrous tissue covered with a modified skin. It also separates the outer ear from the middle ear.

■ BOX 11.4 Middle ear infections

Middle ear infections may be acute or chronic in nature. They are often caused by the spread of microbes from the upper respiratory tract through the pharyngotympanic (auditory) tube. Accumulation of pus in the middle ear can lead to deafness which may be prolonged (glue ear). This can be treated by the insertion of grommets – small plastic tubes inserted through the tympanic membrane which allow for drainage of the middle ear.

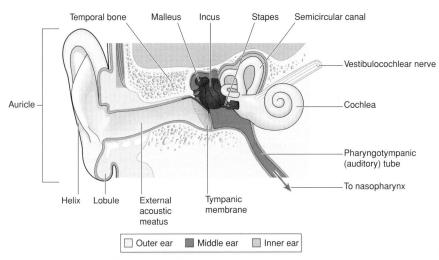

Temporal bone   Malleus   Incus   Stapes   Semicircular canal

Vestibulocochlear nerve

Auricle

Cochlea

Pharyngotympanic
(auditory) tube

To nasopharynx

Helix   Lobule   External   Tympanic
acoustic   membrane
meatus

☐ Outer ear   ■ Middle ear   ☐ Inner ear

Fig. 11.5 The parts of the ear (from Waugh A, Grant A. Ross and Wilson Anatomy and physiology in health and illness. 9th edn. Edinburgh: Churchill Livingstone; 2001).

The middle ear

The middle ear is an irregular space in the temporal bone. It is sometimes called the *tympanic cavity*. It is lined with mucous membrane and contains air, which reaches it through the *pharyngotympanic* or *auditory tube* . The air, at atmospheric pressure, is equal on both sides of the tympanic membrane and allows it to vibrate. The lining of the pharyngotympanic tube is continuous with the nasopharynx.

The tympanic membrane forms the lateral wall of the tympanic cavity. The medial wall separates the middle ear from the inner ear. It is a thin plate of bone in which there are two 'windows'. The *round window* is covered by a membrane which bulges out when the *oval window* moves in. The oval window is occluded by part of one of the *auditory ossicles*.

The auditory ossicles

Three small bones, called the auditory ossicles, extend across the middle ear from the tympanic membrane to the oval window. These bones are shaped like a hammer, an anvil and a stirrup, and are called *malleus, incus* and *stapes*, respectively. The handle of the malleus is in contact with the tympanic membrane and the base of the stapes is in contact with the oval window. The incus lies in between and articulates with the other bones.

The inner ear

The inner ear is a complex arrangement of passages hollowed out of the temporal bone. It is called the *bony labyrinth* and consists of three parts: the *vestibule*, the *semicircular canals* and the *cochlea*. The three semicircular canals open out of the vestibule, which is the part next to the middle ear. The cochlea also opens out of the vestibule. It is shaped like a snail's shell.

The bony labyrinth is full of fluid in which floats the *membranous labyrinth*. The membranous labyrinth is the same shape as the bony labyrinth but

Any movements that affect the inner ear will affect the individual's perception of balance. Movements such as *rocking* affect balance mechanisms in the inner ear, and this in turn elicits parasympathetic responses. Therefore, many soft-tissue manipulations that cause rhythmical movement, and movement therapies, can be very calming.

Music therapy can be used to modify behaviour and mood.

The sense of smell has a more direct impact on the emotions than any of the other senses. In aromatherapy, the odours of essential oils and aromatic plant extracts are used to bring about positive changes in moods. The odours of some essential oils have sedative effects; many can relieve anxiety and facilitate sleep, while others stimulate the mind and improve concentration. Some can even induce a state of mild euphoria.

somewhat smaller. It also contains fluid in which are the hair-like endings of the *vestibulocochlear nerve* (eighth cranial nerve). This nerve has two branches. One branch goes to the cochlea, this is the nerve of hearing. The other, smaller branch supplies the semicircular canals and is concerned with balance.

Hearing and balance

Waves of sound pass into the acoustic meatus and hit the tympanic membrane, which then vibrates. These vibrations are conveyed through the auditory ossicle to the oval window. The oval window vibrates and sets up waves in the fluid in the cochlea. This moves the fluid in the membranous labyrinth and the hair-like nerve endings are simulated. Nervous impulses are generated and are transmitted to the temporal lobe of the cerebral cortex, where they are appreciated as sound and interpreted.

The nerve endings in the semicircular canals are stimulated by the pressure of the fluid changing with the different positions of the head in space. They have nothing to do with hearing but they play some part in maintaining balance.

THE NOSE AND SMELL

The nose

The nose consists of an external and internal portion. The external part is a bony and cartilaginous framework covered with skin which contains many sebaceous glands. The internal portion is a cavity which is divided into a right and left portion by the septum. The roof of the nose consists of a portion of the ethmoid bone which is perforated by small openings that allow branches of the olfactory nerves (sense of smell) to reach the brain (Fig. 11.6).

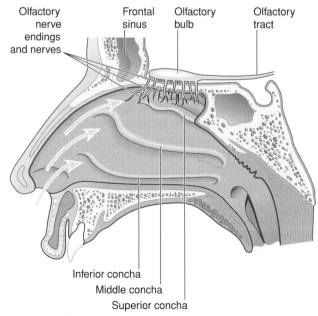

Fig. 11.6 The olfactory structures (from Waugh A, Grant A. Ross and Wilson Anatomy and physiology in health and illness. 9th edn. Edinburgh: Churchill Livingstone; 2001).

The mucosa of the nose has a very rich blood supply which warms inhaled air prior to it descending into the lower respiratory tract. Small hairs help to trap dust and foreign bodies, preventing them from entering the respiratory tract and causing us to cough. Near the roof of the nasal cavity the mucosa turns pale and has a yellowish tint. This is the *olfactory epithelium*, which contains between 10 and 100 million receptors for smell.

Smell

The olfactory nerves (first cranial nerve) carry their information to the brain (thalamus, olfactory centres) for interpretation. Their dendrites and cell bodies lie in the nasal mucosa. Their axons form approximately 20 small bundles which pierce the roof of the nose and end in the olfactory bulbs that lie on the undersurface of the frontal lobes of the cerebral cortex of the brain. The receptors in the olfactory epithelium are very sensitive chemoreceptors and the chemical or gas molecule must first be dissolved in mucus before it can bind to the receptor sites prior to a nervous impulse being generated. These olfactory receptor cells are replaced approximately every month. Bowman's glands are found in the connective tissue that supports the olfactory epithelium, they produce the mucus that is required to dissolve the chemicals and gases in.

Humans have a far less keen sense of smell than animals, and there is a rapid adaptation to smells caused by inhibition of action potentials. Smells can be powerful and can give rise to long-lasting memories, due to their integration and storage into our memories by the limbic system of the brain. Smell and taste are very closely related.

THE SPECIAL SENSES QUESTIONS

Diagrams—Questions 573–593

573–584. The eye

A. Cornea
B. Lacrimal gland
C. Pupil
D. Retina
E. Anterior chamber
F. Vitreous body
G. Lens
H. Ciliary body
I. Conjunctiva
J. Optic nerve
K. Choroid
L. Iris

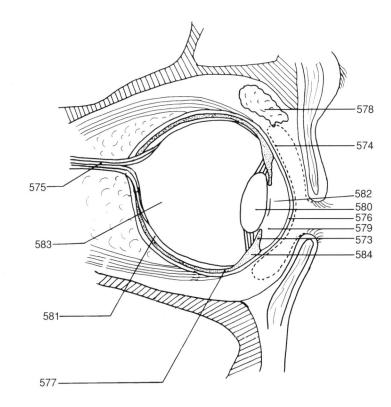

| 573 |
| 574 |
| 575 |
| 576 |
| 577 |
| 578 |
| 579 |
| 580 |
| 581 |
| 582 |
| 583 |
| 584 |

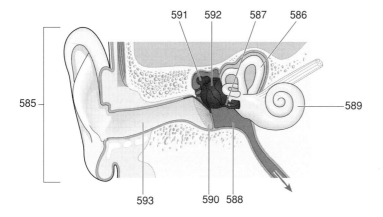

585–593. The ear

A. Auricle
B. External acoustic
    meatus
C. Tympanic
    membrane
D. Middle ear
E. Malleus
F. Incus
G. Stapes
H. Cochlea
 I. Semicircular
    canals

585
586
587
588
589
590
591
592
593

Questions 594–597 are of the multiple choice type

594. The number of muscles attaching each eye to the orbit is: 594
  A. 2
  B. 4
  C. 6
  D. 8.

595. Which one of the following parts of the eyeball is the white part?   595
  A. Cornea
  B. Choroid
  C. Retina
  D. Sclera.

596. The iris is a part of one of the following parts of the eyeball. Which one?   596
  A. Cornea
  B. Choroid
  C. Retina
  D. Sclera.

597. Which one of the following has no refractive power?   597
  A. Aqueous humour
  B. Cornea
  C. Lens
  D. Sclera.

Questions 598–633 are of the true/false type   T | F

598–601. The orbit is:
    598. cone-shaped
    599. spherical
    600. part of the eyeball
    601. part of the skull.

602–605. The lens is:
    602. attached to the ciliary body
    603. biconcave
    604. elastic
    605. transparent.

606–609. Accommodation involves the:
    606. movement of the eye
    607. shape of the lens
    608. size of the pupil
    609. the blind spot.

610–613. The conjunctiva:
    610. covers the front of the eyeball
    611. lines the orbit
    612. lines the eyelids
    613. secretes tears.

614–617. The external acoustic meatus:
    614. lies entirely within the temporal bone
    615. is lined with mucous membrane
    616. is a straight tube
    617. ends at the tympanic membrane.

618–621. The middle ear:
    618. is connected to the nasopharynx
    619. contains the semicircular canals
    620. contains air at atmospheric pressure
    621. contains wax-secreting glands.

622–625. The internal ear:
    622. is a cavity in the temporal bone
    623. is the bony labyrinth
    624. contains the auditory ossicles
    625. contains fluid.

626–629. The cochlea:
    626. consists of three semicircular canals
    627. contains the endings of the vestibulocochlear nerve
    628. is concerned with hearing
    629. is concerned with balance.

630–633. We can hear because: T | F

    630. sounds travel in waves

    631. the incus is in contact with the oval window

    632. pressure is exerted on the nerve endings in the semicircular canals

    633. the tympanic membrane vibrates.

Questions 634–648 are of the matching items type

634–636. From the list on the left select a statement that describes each structure listed on the right.

A. Is composed of voluntary muscle tissue	634. Iris	634
B. Is composed of involuntary muscle tissue	635. Lens	635
C. Is highly elastic	636. Pupil.	636
D. Dilates in dim light		
E. Is attached to the retina		

637–639. From the list on the left select a statement that describes each structure listed on the right.

A. Secretes tears	637. Macula lutea	637
B. Sensitive to dim light	638. Rods	638
C. Part of the choroid	639. Lacrimal gland.	639
D. Consists of cones		
E. Gives stereoscopic vision		

640–642. From the list on the left select the abnormality that results in the conditions on the right.

A. A weak eye muscle	640. Myopia	640
B. An abnormal cornea	641. Cataract	641
C. A detached retina	642. Strabismus.	642
D. Hardening of the lens		
E. An abnormal shaped eyeball		

643–645. From the list on the left select the statement that describes each part of the ear listed on the right.

A. Is made of hyaline cartilage	643. External	643
B. Lies only partly in the temporal bone	644. Internal	644
C. Contains the openings into the pharyngotympanic (auditory) tube	645. Middle.	645
D. Contains the semicircular canals		
E. Contains mastoid air cells		

646–648. From the list on the left select the statement that describes the structures on the right.

A. Is shaped like a stirrup	646. Incus	646
B. Is the middle auditory ossicle	647. Malleus	647
C. Is floating in lymph	648. Stapes.	648
D. Is in contact with the cochlea		
E. Is in contact with the tympanic membrane		

The endocrine system

KEY POINTS

- The pituitary gland
- The thyroid gland
- The parathyroid glands
- The adrenal glands
- The pancreas
- The pineal gland
- The ovaries and testes.

INTRODUCTION

The endocrine glands are distributed throughout the body and play important and diverse roles both in the development and in the everyday functioning of the body. Unlike the sweat and digestive glands, they do not have ducts to carry their secretions to the parts where they are required. The secretions of the endocrine glands go straight into the blood capillaries, hence endocrine glands are called ductless glands. Their secretions are called *hormones*.

The major glands of the endocrine system are:

- pituitary
- thyroid
- parathyroid
- adrenal
- pancreatic islet cells
- pineal
- ovaries and testes.

The gastrointestinal system also secretes hormones (*gastrin* and *secretin*) which act to promote the digestion of food and its movement along the gut.

THE PITUITARY GLAND (HYPOPHYSIS CEREBRI)

The pituitary gland is a small gland about the size and shape of a cherry. It lies in the skull at the base of the brain, to which it is attached (Fig. 12.1). It consists of an anterior and a posterior lobe.

The anterior lobe

The *anterior lobe* produces several hormones, some of which control the activities of other endocrine glands. *Feedback mechanisms* between the anterior pituitary gland and the secretions of these glands ensure that output is regulated and homeostasis maintained. For example, the secretion of *thyroid stimulating hormone* (TSH) which controls the thyroid gland, is

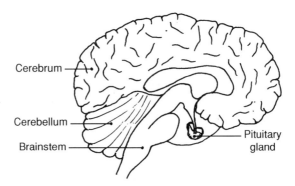

Fig. 12.1 The pituitary gland.

increased if the secretions of thyroid hormones are decreased, and as the thyroid hormones rise, levels of TSH fall (Fig. 12.2).

Other anterior pituitary secretions which control endocrine glands are:

- *adrenocorticotrophic hormone* (ACTH), which controls the cortex of the adrenal glands.
- the *gonadotrophic hormones, luteinizing hormone (LH)* and *follicle stimulating hormone (FSH)*, which control the sex glands.

prolactin is responsible for the initiation and maintenance of lactation in women after childbirth and *growth hormone* affects the growth of cells, including the cells of the epiphyses (the growing section) of long bones.

The posterior lobe

The *posterior lobe* of the pituitary gland produces two hormones, *oxytocin* and *antidiuretic hormone* (also know as *vasopressin*).

Oxytocin is released at the onset of labour, causing contraction of the pregnant uterus. Under the influence of oxytocin, the breasts will secrete milk when the baby starts to suckle (the *suckling reflex*).

Antidiuretic hormone (ADH) controls the amount of water excreted by the kidneys. The more ADH released, the greater the amount of water

---

■ BOX 12.1 Control of growth

In childhood, undersecretion of growth hormone results in stunted growth, although the nervous system (and therefore mental development) is not affected. The condition is called *pituitary dwarfism*. Children with abnormally low secretion may be treated with injections of biosynthetic growth hormone (hGH). A child with oversecretion of growth hormone will grow abnormally tall (*gigantism*).

In adults, too much growth hormone results in thickening of the soft tissues of hands, feet, lips and nose (*acromegaly*) but no gain in height, since *epiphyseal closure* (which occurs in early adulthood) means that the long bones cannot grow any more in length. Excessive secretion of growth hormone may result from a tumour in the pituitary gland.

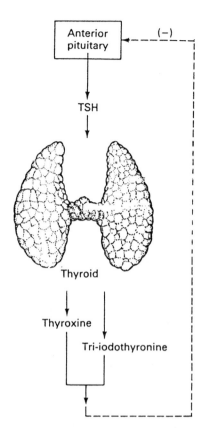

Fig. 12.2 Feedback between the pituitary gland and the thyroid gland (from Hubbard and Methan Physiology for health care students. Edinburgh: Churchill Livingstone; 1987).

reabsorbed from the kidney tubules, and hence the lower the volume of urine produced. Underproduction of ADH (for example following head injury and damage to the pituitary gland) therefore results in excessive loss of fluid from the body, a condition known as *diabetes insipidus*.

THE THYROID GLAND

The thyroid gland (Fig. 12.3) consists of two lobes, one on either side of the larynx, joined by a narrow piece of tissue called the isthmus. It is normally invisible but, if enlarged, it can form an obvious swelling at the base of the neck called a *goitre*.

The thyroid gland consists of numerous follicles held together by connective tissue. It has a very rich blood supply. The follicles contain a fluid called the colloid. Iodine is required in the diet for the proper development of the colloid and the hormones *thyroxine* (T_4) and *tri-iodothyronine* (T_3). These hormones are developed and stored in the colloid for release under the control of thyroid stimulating hormone (TSH) from the anterior pituitary gland.

Thyroxine has many functions. It controls the rate of metabolism and hence body heat production. It is necessary for normal mental and physical development and for healthy hair and skin.

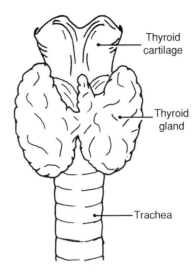

Fig. 12.3 The thyroid gland.

Calcitonin is another hormone released by the 'c-cells' within the thyroid gland. In the presence of calcitonin, blood calcium concentrations fall and less calcium is lost from the bones.

THE PARATHYROID GLANDS

There are four parathyroid glands situated at the back of the thyroid gland. The hormone they produce (*parathyroid hormone* or *PTH*) acts with calcitonin to maintain the correct amount of calcium in the blood and in the bones.

■ **BOX 12.2 Hypothyroidism and hyperthyroidism**

Hypothyroidism in an adult results in a reduced metabolic rate, leading to sensitivity to cold, lethargy and a slow pulse. The skin becomes coarse and puffy and the hair dry. The condition is called *myxoedema* and is treated with oral thyroxine.

In the developing fetus and in children, hypothyroidism results in slow growth and may result in permanent brain damage since the thyroid hormones are required for normal mental development. This is called *congenital hypothyroidism*. Fortunately, it can be detected by means of routine screening carried out in all newborn babies. It is treatable with oral thyroxine.

An overactive thyroid gland (*hyperthyroidism*) produces an overactive individual. The metabolic rate is increased so that energy is burnt up and the individual may lose weight and feel warm all the time. Pulse rate is increased and the person may feel nervous and excitable. In some cases the eyes may protrude (*exophthalmos*). There are various treatments for patients with hyperthyroidism: drugs that inhibit the uptake of iodine by the gland, radioactive iodine which will destroy the cells of the gland, or surgical removal of the gland.

In the presence of PTH, blood calcium concentrations rise as more calcium is released from the bones. If these glands are overactive, the amount of calcium in the blood is raised, causing thirst, polyuria (increased volume of urine) and tiredness. The bones may become painful and easily fractured. Undersecretion of the hormone results in a lowered blood calcium which may lead to muscular spasms (tetany) and possibly convulsions.

THE ADRENAL OR SUPRARENAL GLANDS

There are two adrenal glands, one situated above each kidney. These glands consist of two parts, a cortex on the outside and a medulla in the centre.

The adrenal cortex

A number of different hormones are secreted by the adrenal cortex. They are called *adrenal steroids* and include *cortisol* and *aldosterone*. The function of cortisol is to regulate carbohydrate metabolism. In times of stress, this steroid converts protein and fat into glucose, and raises blood pressure. Aldosterone regulates sodium and potassium balance and, if aldosterone secretion is too low, excessive loss of sodium results in severe dehydration.

Oversecretion of the adrenal cortex (or excessive use of steroid drugs) therefore leads to a range of disorders of energy and salt and water storage, a condition called *Cushing's syndrome*. Excess salt and water reabsorbed leads to oedema and high blood pressure, fat deposition on the trunk and the face is increased, and the skin becomes thinner (Fig. 12.4).

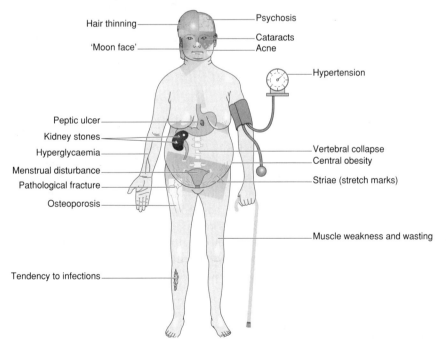

Fig. 12.4 The systemic features of Cushing's syndrome (from Waugh A, Grant A. Ross and Wilson Anatomy and physiology in health and illness. 9th edn. Edinburgh: Churchill Livingstone; 2001).

If prolonged stress disrupts homeostatic mechanisms, some of the hormones, e.g. the 'fight or flight' hormones of the adrenal medulla and the glucocorticoids of the adrenal cortex, may produce detrimental effects. These include suppression of the immune system, sleep disturbances, digestive problems, etc. Complementary therapies and stress reduction regimes may help restore balance, and reduce the magnitude of the stress response.

■ BOX 12.3 Allergies, inflammation and the immune system

The adrenal steroids such as cortisol (hydrocortisone), and synthetic steroid drugs such as prednisolone, suppress allergic reactions and reduce inflammation. They are therefore used as drugs in the treatment of conditions such as eczema, asthma and rheumatoid arthritis. In higher doses these drugs reduce immune responses, so they may be given to a patient who has received a tissue or organ transplant, to reduce the risk of rejection of the transplant.

Undersecretion of the adrenal cortex is called *Addison's disease*. In this condition the patient has low blood pressure, there is loss of sodium and water from the body and the patient develops muscle weakness, nausea and vomiting.

The other hormones from the adrenal cortex are the sex hormones – *testosterone, oestrogen* and *progesterone*. Oversecretion of these hormones in a young child may lead to changes in sexual development.

The adrenal medulla

The medulla of the adrenal gland produces *adrenaline* and *noradrenaline*. These hormones work in conjunction with the sympathetic nervous system. Adrenaline causes the blood pressure and pulse rate to rise, breathing becomes more rapid and extra glucose is liberated from the stores in the liver. This is the 'flight or fight' response which arises when the body is confronted by an immediate stress and acts to prepare the body to respond quickly. The release of adrenaline into the blood is accompanied by increased stimulation of the sympathetic nervous system, described in Chapter 10.

THE PANCREAS

A specialized group of cells, called the *islets of Langerhans*, in the pancreas acts as an endocrine gland. *Insulin*, from beta cells, and *glucagon*, from alpha cells, regulate blood glucose levels. In the presence of insulin, blood glucose concentrations fall, as more glucose is taken up by cells and storage of glucose is increased. Glucagon has the opposite effect, namely, blood glucose levels rise as more glucose is released from stores. The release of insulin and glucagon is regulated by blood glucose concentrations. If blood glucose falls, more glucagon is released, if glucose levels rise, more insulin is released. In this way, blood glucose concentrations can be kept fairly constant between meals.

Patient education plays an important part in the treatment of diabetes mellitus. This is often undertaken by a specialist diabetes nurse. For example, patients with type I diabetes learn to monitor their own blood glucose level, to administer their own injections of insulin, and to recognize the symptoms of hypoglycaemia. The importance of diet in controlling type 2 diabetes is also stressed.

THE PINEAL GLAND

This is a small gland situated in the brain. It secretes a hormone called *melatonin* which, in seasonally breeding mammals, is responsible for

■ **BOX 12.4 Diabetes mellitus**

This is the most commonly encountered endocrine disorder. It occurs because of the lack of production of insulin by the islet cells (type 1) or due to resistance of cells to insulin (type 2). Type 1 diabetes mellitus is more often diagnosed in younger people and results in loss of weight, excessive thirst and the production of large volumes of urine. In the absence of treatment, fats are broken down by the body and this may result in a life-threatening condition in which the blood becomes more acidic, called *acidosis*. Type 1 diabetics have to replace insulin by self-administered injections of the hormone twice or more times a day.

Type 2 diabetics (the more common type) may not recognize they have the condition until a routine blood test reveals high blood glucose concentrations. In some of these patients, weight loss is all that is needed to restore sensitivity to insulin. Others may take oral drugs to reduce their blood glucose levels.

Despite many advances in the control of diabetes mellitus, there are long-term effects of the disease which result in damage to the circulation. Diabetics are therefore at greater risk of suffering from heart disease, kidney disease and loss of vision.

timing of the biological clock. In humans, melatonin secretion increases during the hours of darkness, but its functions are not yet completely understood.

THE OVARIES

The ovaries are the female sex glands and will be described in Chapter 13. They secrete the hormones that bring about the physiological changes which occur in a girl at puberty, and they maintain the normal menstrual cycle in a woman during her childbearing years.

THE TESTES

The testes are the male sex glands. The hormone *testosterone* is responsible for the changes occurring in a boy at puberty and for maintaining the normal reproductive functioning of the adult male.

Endocrine system questions

Questions 649–652 are of the multiple choice type

649. Which of the following is a feature of hypothyroidism?   649
  A. Nervous tension
  B. Weight loss
  C. Exophthalmus
  D. Lethargy.

650. Which of the following is a feature of hyperthyroidism?   650
  A. Bradycardia
  B. Raised metabolic rate
  C. Feeling cold
  D. Coarse hair.

651. Which of the following is a feature of undersecretion of the parathyroid glands?   651
  A. Soft bones
  B. Fractures
  C. Tetany
  D. Increased metabolic rate.

652. Which of the following is a feature of undersecretion of insulin?   652
  A. Gigantism
  B. Tetany
  C. Weight gain
  D. Increased thirst.

Questions 653–684 are of the true/false type

T | F

653–656. The pituitary gland:
653. is attached to the brain
654. has four lobes
655. controls growth
656. controls other endocrine glands.

657–660. Anti-diuretic hormone:
657. is secreted by the posterior lobe of the pituitary gland
658. controls blood glucose
659. raises blood pressure
660. influences the breast to produce milk.

661–664. Thyroxine:
661. requires iodine for its production
662. is stored in a colloid
663. controls metabolism
664. influences mental development.

665–668. The adrenal cortex:
665. is the inner part of the adrenal gland
666. produces adrenaline
667. regulates carbohydrate metabolism
668. is controlled by the anterior pituitary gland.

669–672. The parathyroid glands:
669. are situated next to the pituitary gland
670. secrete calcitonin
671. secrete melatonin
672. regulate blood calcium.

673–676 Insulin:
673. is secreted by the alpha cells of the islets of Langerhans
674. breaks down glucose
675. is secreted in excess in diabetes mellitus
676. is used to treat diabetes mellitus.

677–680. Cortisol:
677. is secreted by the adrenal cortex
678. is a steroid
679. if secreted in excess, results in Addison's disease
680. regulates blood calcium.

681–684. Adrenaline:
681. is a steroid
682. may be used to treat inflammation
683. acts in conjunction with the sympathetic nervous system
684. increases heart rate.

Complete the following paragraph using words from the following list:

A. beta   685
B. alpha   686
C. pancreas   687
D. liver   688
E. lowering   689
F. rise   690
G. urine
H. insulin
 I. glucose
 J. cortisol

'The [685] cells of the islets of Langerhans in the [686] secrete a hormone, insulin, which is responsible for [687] blood glucose levels by promoting uptake of glucose into cells. In the absence of insulin, blood glucose levels [688] and the patient suffers from weight loss and increased excretion of [689] which contains glucose. The treatment for this type of diabetes mellitus is the injection of [690]'.

The reproductive system

13

CELL DIVISION

Single-celled organisms such as bacteria reproduce by simply dividing into two. The parent cell grows and matures until the time comes for it to divide. The two resulting daughter cells are exact replicas of the parent. Human beings, like many other multicellular organisms, reproduce by means of sexual reproduction rather than simple cell division.

In sexual reproduction two *gametes*, one from the female and one from the male, fuse to form a *zygote*. Human gametes are called ova (from the woman) and spermatozoa (from the man). The formation of gametes involves a specialized cell division called *meiosis*, which results in cells with half the normal number of chromosomes. Meiosis only takes place in the ovaries and testes, i.e. the gonads. It must occur in the formation of gametes so that on fusion of an ovum and a spermatozoon, the resulting zygote has the normal number of chromosomes. The zygote then develops into a fetus. In human cells there are 46 chromosomes in the nucleus of each cell. In the process of meiosis, ova and spermatozoa are produced, each with 23 chromosomes in the nucleus (Fig. 13.1). When these two cells unite, the resulting zygote will therefore contain the normal 46 chromosomes and inherits half its chromosomes from the mother and half from the father.

The sex of the child depends on the sex chromosomes. Within the 23 chromosomes in each gamete, there is one sex chromosome, either an X or a Y chromosome. A zygote which inherits two X chromosomes will develop into a girl, a boy is the result of an X and a Y chromosome. Figure 13.2 indicates how division of the sex chromosomes into the gametes will result in equal proportions of male and female zygotes and hence a balance of males to females.

The reproductive systems of male and female animals consist of internal and external organs (i.e. the external genitalia), all of which are designed to enable sexual reproduction, and subsequent development of the fetus, to occur. Secondary sexual characteristics are changes associated with sexual maturity, for example, changes in fat deposition and breast development in women, facial hair growth and lowering of the voice in men. These characteristics are the result of secretion of hormones from the maturing gonads.

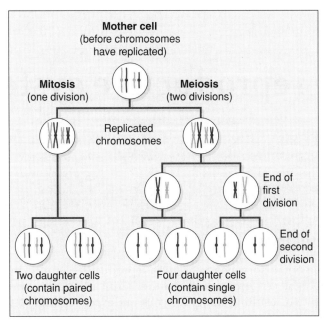

Fig. 13.1 Meiosis.

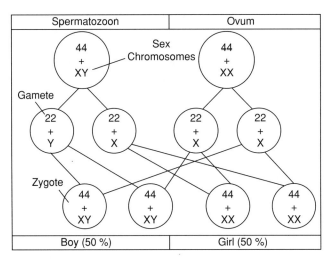

Fig. 13.2 Division of the sex chromosomes at meiosis.

THE FEMALE REPRODUCTIVE SYSTEM

The ovaries

The ovaries are the female gonads or sex glands. They produce the ova and also the sex hormones oestrogen and progesterone. They do not begin to function until a girl reaches puberty at the age of 12–14 years.

The ovaries are small, almond-shaped glands, about 2–3 cm long. They are situated in the pelvic cavity, one on either side of the uterus (Fig. 13.3).

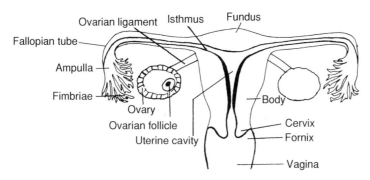

Fig. 13.3 Female reproductive system.

They consist of two layers, the outer cortex and the inner medulla, which is composed of fibrous tissue.

The cortex of the ovary contains the ovarian *follicles*. Each ovarian follicle contains fluid and an immature ovum. At puberty and every 28 days from then until the menopause (about 50 years of age) one follicle expels its mature ovum into a uterine or *Fallopian tube*. If sexual intercourse takes place at this time, fertilization may occur (in the Fallopian tube) and the resulting zygote then passes to the uterus where development to a fetus may follow. After the follicle has ruptured and expelled its ovum, it becomes the *corpus luteum*, which remains throughout pregnancy. If pregnancy does not occur, the corpus luteum degenerates and becomes a fibrous scar on the surface of the ovary. The lining of the uterus is shed (menstruation) and the cycle starts again with development of another follicle (see The menstrual cycle, below).

The ovary produces the female sex hormones oestrogen and progesterone; oestrogen comes from the ovarian follicle and progesterone from the corpus luteum. At puberty, oestrogen is responsible for the development of secondary sexual characteristics, such as growth of the breasts, and with each menstrual cycle the hormones prepare the uterus for implantation and pregnancy.

The uterus

The uterus is a hollow organ about 10 cm long. It is situated in the pelvic cavity between the rectum and the bladder (Fig. 13.4). Projecting from it on either side are the two Fallopian or uterine tubes.

The uterus has a thick muscular coat (*myometrium*), which consists of smooth muscle. Myometrium is therefore controlled by the autonomic nervous system and its contractions are not under voluntary control. The non-pregnant uterus is pear shaped but in pregnancy the myometrium must stretch and expand to accommodate the growing fetus. The broad upper part lying between the uterine tubes is the *fundus*. The main part is called the body. This narrows to form the *cervix* or neck which projects down into the *vagina*. The opening from the body into the cervix is the *internal os* and the opening into the vagina is the *external os*.

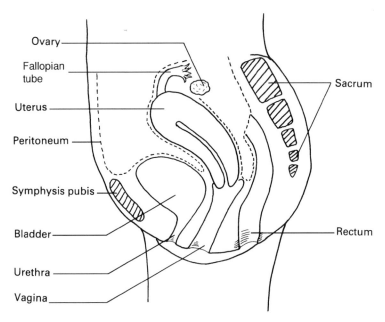

Fig. 13.4 Female pelvic organs.

The uterus and uterine tubes are covered by a fold of the *peritoneum* called the *broad ligament*. The broad ligament and the *round ligament*, which extends from the uterus to the vulva, hold the uterus in a position of *ante-version* and *anteflexion*. This means that it leans forwards and is bent almost at right angles over the bladder.

The uterus is lined with a mucous membrane called the *endometrium*. The blood supply is from the uterine artery, a branch of the iliac artery.

The fallopian tubes are lined with *ciliated epithelium*, the cilia help move the ovum along the tube towards the uterus. The ends of the tubes near the ovaries have fringe-like projections called *fimbriae*. These pass through the posterior fold of the broad ligament into the peritoneal cavity and one long fimbria lies near the corresponding ovary. The wide part of the fallopian tube is the *ampulla*, the narrow part of the tube leading to the uterus is called the *isthmus*.

The vagina

The vagina is the passage leading from the uterus to the external organs. It is a flattened, muscular tube lined with *stratified squamous epithelium*. Where the cervix enters the vagina is the *fornix*. The exit of the vagina is in the vulva behind the urethral orifice. The *hymen* is the membrane (with no known function) which, in some girls, partially covers the vaginal opening.

The vulva or external genitalia

The term vulva covers all parts of the external genitals. The *labia majora* are two thick folds of skin and fat on which coarse hair grows at the onset of puberty. Lying between them are the *labia minora*, two smaller folds of skin

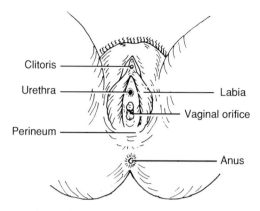

Fig. 13.5 Female external genitalia.

Clitoris

Urethra

Perineum

Labia

Vaginal orifice

Anus

containing many sebaceous glands. Where these folds meet anteriorly is the *clitoris*, which corresponds to the penis in the male (Fig. 13.5).

The vestibule between the labia minora is where the vaginal and urethral orifices are situated. The vestibular glands secrete mucus which lubricates the vagina.

THE MENSTRUAL CYCLE

From puberty to the menopause a series of changes occur in the uterus, usually every 28 days. This is called the *menstrual cycle* (Fig. 13.6). It is controlled by the ovarian hormones which, in turn, are stimulated by the *gonadotrophic hormones* (*luteinizing hormone* or *LH* and *follicle stimulating hormone* or *FSH*) from the anterior lobe of the pituitary gland.

The menstrual period, which is the shedding of the endometrium by the uterus, lasts for about 5 days. For the next 9 days, under the influence of follicle stimulating hormone secreted by the anterior pituitary gland, the ovarian follicles secrete oestrogen which repairs the uterine lining and causes the endometrium to thicken. Around the fourteenth day ovulation takes place. A follicle bursts and liberates a mature ovum. The secretion of

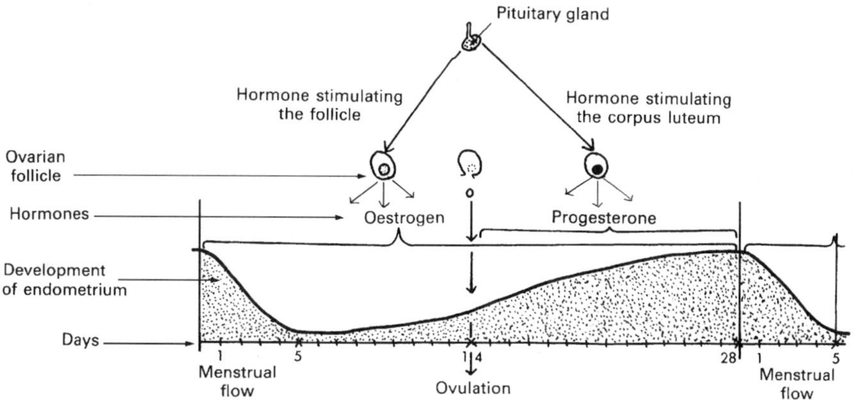

Exposure of a fetus to *rubella* or German measles can result in permanent damage, so checking that antibodies are present in the maternal circulation (a blood sample is needed) is a step women can take if they are planning to become pregnant. Maternal intake of folic acid is also important, a diet low in this vitamin can lead to *neural tube defects* such as *spina bifida*. Women are recommended to ensure their diet has enough of this vitamin leading up to conception and in early pregnancy.

As soon as pregnancy is confirmed, the mother is invited to attend a booking clinic where she will meet the midwife who will be seeing her through pregnancy. In most cases, the midwife is the first point of call for the mother, monitoring changes through the pregnancy and taking urine and blood samples for analysis when appropriate. ABO blood grouping and rhesus factor are established, since this is relevant if the mother is rhesus negative. The mother's blood haemoglobin level is also checked. Blood tests are also available to give estimates of risk of congenital conditions such as Down's syndrome.

Pituitary gland

Hormone stimulating the follicle

Hormone stimulating the corpus luteum

Ovarian follicle

Hormones

Oestrogen

Progesterone

Development of endometrium

Days

1   5

Menstrual flow

14

Ovulation

28 1   5

Menstrual flow

Fig. 13.6 The menstrual cycle.

■ BOX 13.1 Menstrual problems

Amenorrhoea means no menstruation. In non-pregnant women of childbearing age, this is not normal and indicates lack of ovulation. *Oligomenorrhoea* refers to few menstrual periods. *Dysmenorrhoea* is when menstruation is associated with excessive pain, and *menorrhagia* refers to excessive blood loss at menstruation. All of these conditions are often treatable, sometimes with hormone preparations. Underlying causes should be investigated; for example, excessive spread of endometrial tissue (*endometriosis*) outside the normal confines of the uterus, can lead to unusual bleeding and menstrual pain.

Premenstrual syndrome (PMS) is a condition experienced by many women in the days leading up to menstruation. Symptoms include mood changes (irritability, depression), feeling bloated and breast enlargement.

Anecdotal evidence suggests that both reflexology and aromatherapy can be helpful in regulating the menstrual cycle and relieving some menstrual problems, such as dysmenorrhoea and menorrhagia.

Symptoms of PMS, such as bloating and irritability, can be relieved by massage and the use of essential oils.

Anecdotal evidence would also suggest that some of the distressing symptoms of the menopause could also be relieved by aromatherapy and reflexology.

luteinizing hormone from the anterior pituitary gland stimulates the secretion of progesterone from the ruptured follicle, which is now called the corpus luteum. Progesterone causes the endometrium to thicken and a watery mucus is produced. This is preparing the uterus to receive a fertilized ovum.

If fertilization takes place, progesterone continues to be secreted, firstly by the corpus luteum and then by the placenta, and the menstrual cycle stops for the duration of pregnancy. If fertilization does not occur, the corpus luteum ceases to function and the endometrium is shed. This debris passes out of the uterus via the vagina in the form of a discharge of blood and dead cells. The secretion of FSH rises again and another follicle is destined to develop to ovulation. The first day of the next cycle has begun.

FERTILIZATION TO BIRTH

The fertilization of the human ovum by the spermatozoon occurs in the ampulla of a Fallopian tube. Twins and triplets are the result of fertilization of two or three ova, although in humans ovulation of a single ovum is the norm. The resulting zygote starts to divide by mitosis and forms a ball of cells called a *morula*. The morula develops into a *blastocyst* as fluid accumulates in the centre of the clump. Four to five days after fertilization, the blastocyst reaches the uterus, where implantation into the uterine wall will occur, and the placenta develops. This will allow transfer of oxygen and nutrients to the growing embryo, which by 8 weeks has assumed the shape of the human being. By 12 weeks the embryo is referred to as a fetus. The gestation period in humans is, by convention, counted from the time of the last menstrual period before conception and is taken to be 40 weeks. During this time the fetus grows and develops until it is capable of a separate existence.

Rarely, implantation of the fertilized ovum occurs outside the uterus, for example in a Fallopian tube. This is termed an *ectopic pregnancy*.

■ **BOX 13.2 Infertility**

The process of reproduction is complex and it is not surprising that there are plenty of opportunities for events to go wrong. In approximately one-third of cases of infertility no identifiable cause is discovered and in the remaining cases the cause is equally likely to be of male or female origin.

Male infertility may arise due to lack of production of spermatozoa, lack of motility or inability to ejaculate. Spermatozoa production will only proceed at temperatures below that of the body core, fertility will therefore be affected if the testes do not descend (hence checks undertaken in young boys to ensure the testes have descended into the scrotum), or in conditions where the testes are subjected to heat.

The spermatozoa must also demonstrate normal motility and the ability to penetrate the cervical mucus in the female partner. There are techniques for overcoming low spermatozoa counts, some of these techniques involve extracting spermatozoa from the seminal fluid and injecting them into an ovum in laboratory conditions. The fertilized ovum is then replaced in the female reproductive system.

A failure to ejaculate may be caused by psychological of physiological problems. A blockage in the vas deferens or ejaculatory ducts would prevent conception.

Impotence means an inability to sustain an erection for sufficient time to perform sexual intercourse, drugs are available to help in the treatment.

Infertility in the woman often results from lack of ovulation. Not all menstrual cycles result in release of a mature ovum. Drugs can be used to increase the chance of ovulation, but one side-effect is the chance of multiple ovulation and hence multiple births.

Salpingitis is inflammation of the Fallopian tubes. This may result in blockage of the tubes and hence infertility.

At the end of gestation, changes in the hormonal environment (including secretion of *oxytocin* from the mother's posterior pituitary gland) result in the smooth muscle of the uterus going through a series of involuntary contractions. The connective tissue of the cervix softens and the cervix dilates. This process is known as *labour* and it results in the expulsion first of the fetus and then of the placenta.

THE MAMMARY GLANDS

The mammary glands, or breasts, are accessory glands of the female reproductive system. They are present in both sexes but only develop in the female.

The breasts develop at puberty, when they are influenced by the ovarian hormones, particularly oestrogen. They only function after the birth of a child, when they are stimulated to produce milk by *prolactin* from the pituitary gland. The release of milk is then stimulated by the act of the baby suckling, which prompts secretion of oxytocin from the posterior pituitary gland. The return of the uterus to its pre-pregnant state is thus promoted by the infant suckling, as oxytocin also stimulates contraction of the stretched myometrium.

Each breast consists of a number of lobes with ducts which reach the surface at the nipple. These ducts are called the lactiferous ducts. They are supported by fibrous tissue and fat. The amount of adipose tissue determines the size of the breasts.

THE MALE REPRODUCTIVE SYSTEM

The male reproductive system is responsible for the production of spermatozoan, or male germ cells, and for projecting them into the female vagina. The spermatozoa are small cells with long tails. The tail gives the cell mobility and drives it up through the uterus into the fallopian tubes where it may fuse with an ovum. Millions of these cells are liberated at ejaculation. The male genital organs are the *testes*, the *vas deferens* and *ejaculatory ducts*, the *penis*, the *seminal vesicles* and the *prostate gland* (Fig. 13.7).

The testes

The testes are the glands that produce the spermatozoa and the male sex hormone testosterone. Testosterone produces the characteristic changes in a boy at puberty. The secretion of testosterone and the development of spermatozoa are stimulated by follicle stimulating hormone and luteinizing hormone secreted by the anterior lobe of the pituitary gland.

Puberty occurs later in boys than in girls. The boy is between 13 to 16 years old before his voice breaks, hair grows on his face and body and the external genitalia enlarge. At this time the testes are activated to produce spermatozoa.

The testes develop in the fetus on the posterior wall of the abdomen and they descend into the *scrotum*, a sac of thin, dark-coloured skin behind the penis, before birth. They descend through the *inguinal canal* in the groin, carrying with them part of the peritoneum which remains as a covering. They also carry with them the ducts, the blood vessels and the nerves.

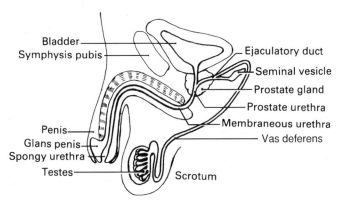

Fig. 13.7 Male reproductive system.

These structures form the spermatic cords which suspend the testes in the scrotum. The position of the testes in the scrotum ensures the best conditions for sperm production, i.e. below the core body temperature. Undescended testes is one cause of male infertility.

Each testis consists of 200 or 300 lobules. Each lobule contains several convoluted tubules in which the spermatozoa are produced. Between the tubules are the interstitial cells which secrete testosterone. From the tubules the developing spermatozoa pass through a series of twisted ducts into the vas deferens, which carries them up through the spermatic cord into the pelvis.

The seminal vesicles

The seminal vesicles are two small sacs which lie at the back of the bladder. The lining of these structures secretes a fluid called *seminal fluid* which helps to nourish the spermatozoa. Each seminal vesicle has a short duct which joins up with the corresponding vas deferens to form the *ejaculatory ducts*. The ejaculatory ducts pass through the prostate gland and join the urethra.

The prostate gland

The prostate gland produces a thin lubricating fluid. It lies at the base of the bladder and surrounds the urethra. This gland may become enlarged in old age, when it will obstruct the urethra, causing acute retention of urine.

The penis

The penis is the common passage for *semen* and urine. Semen is the fluid ejaculate which contains spermatozoa and seminal fluid derived from the seminal vesicles and prostate gland. About 3 ml of semen are ejaculated at orgasm, and this contains about 300 million sperm. A normal sperm count would be between 60 to 100 million spermatozoa/ml, anything less than 40 million spermatozoa/ml is called *oligospermia* and will reduce fertility.

The urethra is about 20 cm long. There are two urethral sphincter muscles. The internal sphincter lies at the neck of the bladder and the external sphincter is in the membranous part of the urethra.

The penis consists of three columns of *erectile tissue* and involuntary muscle tissue covered with skin. It has a rich blood supply and when engorged with blood it becomes enlarged and erect. The tip of the penis is a bulbous structure called the *glans penis*. This is partially covered by a fold of skin called the *prepuce*. The prepuce or foreskin should be loose. If tight it may have to be cut, an operation called *circumcision*.

REPRODUCTION AND AGEING

Although the production of spermatozoa continues into old age, prostatic enlargement or *hyperplasia* affects 80% of men by the time they reach the age of 80. This results in poor bladder emptying as the urethra is compressed. If untreated, urine may be retained to the extent that the bladder capacity is exceeded, and 'back pressure' on the kidneys can lead to kidney damage. Urinary retention must be treated swiftly. Prostatic enlargement is operable, and does not always result from cancer.

Although there are records of men becoming fathers in their eighties, fertility in women declines as they approach their forties. The release of ova (and hence menstrual cycles) becomes less frequent, ceasing altogether at the *menopause*, after which fertilization is not possible. In Western societies the average age at menopause is 50. The reason for the loss of fertility in women is that female babies are born with a finite number of follicles in their ovaries. By the age of 50, these follicles have disappeared and not only are there no more ova present, but the main source of oestrogen (the follicles) has also gone. The loss of oestrogen is associated with menopausal symptoms, which include hot flushes and mood swings, which in some women may last a few years while the hormonal environment re-adjusts.

REPRODUCTIVE SYSTEM QUESTIONS

Diagrams—Questions 691–721

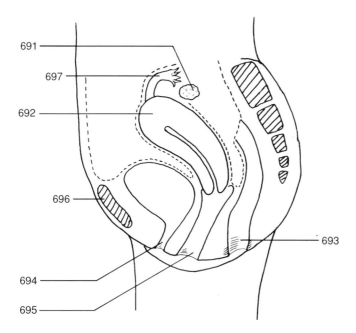

691–697. The female reproductive system

A. Uterus
B. Vagina
C. Ovary
D. Fallopian tube
E. Urethra
F. Rectum
G. Symphysis pubis

| 691 |
| 692 |
| 693 |
| 694 |
| 695 |
| 696 |
| 697 |

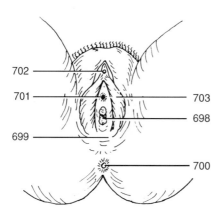

698–703. The external female genitalia

A. Anus
B. Clitoris
C. Labia
D. Perineum
E. Vaginal orifice
F. Urethral orifice

| 698 |
| 699 |
| 700 |
| 701 |
| 702 |
| 703 |

704–713. The uterus and ovaries

A. Fundus
B. Body
C. Fornix
D. Fallopian tube
E. Cervix
F. Endometrium
G. Fimbriae
H. Ampulla
 I. Mature ovarian
    follicle
J. Ovary

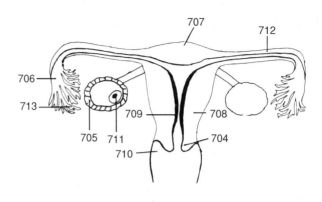

| 704 |
| 705 |
| 706 |
| 707 |
| 708 |
| 709 |
| 710 |
| 711 |
| 712 |
| 713 |

714–721. Male reproductive organs

A. Prostate gland
B. Seminal vesicles
C. Scrotum
D. Testes
E. Vas deferens
F. Symphysis pubis
G. Glans penis
H. Bladder

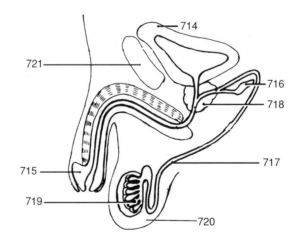

| 714 |
| 715 |
| 716 |
| 717 |
| 718 |
| 719 |
| 720 |
| 721 |

Questions 722–728 are of the multiple choice type

722. The menstrual cycle: 722
  A. relies on ovarian hormones LH and FSH
  B. is approximately 14 days long
  C. starts on the day of ovulation
  D. begins at menopause.

723. Which one of the following is a characteristic of the corpus luteum? It: 723
  A. contains the mature ovum
  B. secretes progesterone
  C. is not influenced by the pituitary gland
  D. becomes the ovarian follicle.

724. Which of the following cells has only 23 chromosomes?   724
  A. A fertilized ovum
  B. An ordinary body cell
  C. A gamete
  D. Any of the cells of the embryo.

725. On which one of the following days of the menstrual cycle does ovulation occur?   725
  A. 5th
  B. 10th
  C. 14th
  D. 28th.

726. About which week of gestation does the embryo become a fetus?   726
  A. 4
  B. 12
  C. 16
  D. 32.

727. Which one of the following is a function of the vas deferens? It: 727
  A. carries semen to the penis
  B. carries spermatozoa to the seminal vesicles
  C. carries testosterone to the bloodstream
  D. is a common passage for urine and semen.

728. The interstitial cells of the testes secrete one of the following: 728
  A. FSH
  B. Semen
  C. Spermatozoa
  D. Testosterone.

Questions 729–756 are of the true/false type   T | F

729–732. The uterus:
   729. lies inside the peritoneal cavity
   730. is covered by the peritoneum
   731. lies posterior to the bladder
   732. lies in a position of anteversion.

733–736. The fallopian tubes:
   733. are broadest where they leave the uterus
   734. are lined with ciliated epithelium
   735. consist of ampulla and isthmus
   736. are the site of fertilization.

737–740. The ovaries:
   737. are pelvic organs
   738. release many ova at each menstrual cycle
   739. cease to release ova at the menopause
   740. are the source of FSH and LH.

741–744. The ovarian follicles:
   741. contain the ova
   742. secrete oestrogen
   743. secrete progesterone
   744. become the corpus luteum.

745–748. The testes
   745. are covered by part of the peritoneum
   746. develop in the abdomen
   747. consist of two lobules
   748. are contained in the scrotum.

749–752. Semen contains:
   749. spermatozoa
   750. seminal fluid
   751. testosterone
   752. prostatic fluid.

753–756. Prostatic enlargement:
   753. is a common condition in older men
   754. always indicates cancer
   755. may lead to retention of urine
   756. may lead to kidney damage.

Answers

CHAPTER 1—CELLS, TISSUES AND SYSTEMS

Diagrams

1—C	6—E	11—B	16—D
2—B	7—G	12—D	17—F
3—E	8—H	13—I	18—B
4—A	9—A	14—F	19—E
5—D	10—C	15—A	20—C

Multiple choice

21—B	25—B	29—D	33—B
22—B	26—C	30—C	34—A
23—B	27—B	31—C	35—B
24—D	28—C	32—C	

CHAPTER 2—THE SKELETAL SYSTEM

Diagrams

36—C	49—C	62—C	75—D
37—E	50—D	63—E	76—A
38—A	51—A	64—D	77—D
39—B	52—G	65—A	78—E
40—D	53—F	66—B	79—C
41—D	54—C	67—C	80—B
42—A	55—E	68—B	81—E
43—C	56—B	69—A	82—F
44—B	57—D	70—D	83—A
45—F	58—D	71—E	84—C
46—A	59—A	72—B	85—B
47—E	60—C	73—C	86—D
48—B	61—B	74—A	

Multiple choice

87—C	90—C	92—D	94—B
88—B	91—D	93—A	95—A
89—B			

True/false

96—T	100—F	104—F	108—F
97—F	101—T	105—T	109—F
98—F	102—F	106—T	110—T
99—T	103—T	107—F	111—T

Matching items

112—D	115—A	117—D	119—A
113—C	116—B	118—D	120—E
114—E			

CHAPTER 3—THE JOINTS

Diagrams

121—B	122—C	123—A	124—D

Multiple choice

125—C	127—A	129—C	130—C
126—C	128—B		

Matching items

131—C	133—D	135—A	136—B
132—B	134—E		

CHAPTER 4—THE MUSCLES

Diagrams

137—A	141—H	144—A	147—C
138—C	142—E	145—B	148—G
139—D	143—D	146—F	149—I
140—B			

Multiple choice

150—D	151—C

True/false

152—T	157—T	162—F	167—T
153—F	158—F	163—T	168—F
154—T	159—T	164—T	169—T
155—F	160—T	165—F	170—F
156—T	161—F	166—T	171—T

Matching items

172—E	173—C	174—B

CHAPTER 5—THE CIRCULATORY SYSTEM

Diagrams

175—E	181—D	186—E	191—E

176—B	182—G	187—C	192—G
177—G	183—A	188—F	193—F
178—F	184—B	189—B	194—D
179—A	185—D	190—C	195—A
180—C			

Multiple choice

196—B	199—C	202—C	204—D
197—B	200—A	203—B	205—C
198—B	201—C		

True/false

206—T	218—F	230—T	242—F
207—F	219—T	231—T	243—T
208—T	220—T	232—F	244—T
209—F	221—F	233—F	245—T
210—F	222—F	234—T	246—F
211—F	223—T	235—T	247—T
212—T	224—T	236—F	248—F
213—T	225—T	237—T	249—T
214—T	226—T	238—T	250—T
215—T	227—F	239—T	251—F
216—T	228—T	240—T	252—F
217—F	229—F	241—F	253—F

Matching items

254—D	257—C	260—E	263—D
255—B	258—D	261—C	264—A
256—C	259—E	262—A	265—E

CHAPTER 6—THE RESPIRATORY SYSTEM

Diagrams

266—B	270—F	273—D	276—C
267—D	271—A	274—A	277—B
268—G	272—C	275—E	278—F
269—E			

Multiple choice

279—B	281—D	283—B	285—C
280—B	282—C	284—B	286—D

True/false

287—F	295—T	303—F	311—T
288—T	296—F	304—F	312—F
289—F	297—F	305—F	313—F
290—T	298—T	306—T	314—F
291—T	299—F	307—F	315—T

292—F	300—T	308—T	316—F
293—T	301—F	309—T	317—T
294—F	302—T	310—F	318—T

Matching items

319—E	321—D	323—B	324—D
320—B	322—C		

CHAPTER 7—THE DIGESTIVE SYSTEM

Diagrams

325—F	332—E	338—B	344—F
326—G	333—G	339—A	345—B
327—A	334—C	340—C	346—C
328—D	335—D	341—E	347—E
329—B	336—A	342—B	348—A
330—C	337—F	343—D	349—D
331—E			

Multiple choice

350—D	352—D	354—B	356—D
351—B	353—B	355—B	357—A

True/false

358—T	363—F	368—T	373—T
359—F	364—T	369—T	374—F
360—T	365—T	370—F	375—F
361—T	366—F	371—T	376—T
362—T	367—T	372—F	377—F

Matching items

378—E	381—C	384—E	387—B
379—D	382—E	385—D	388—D
380—B	383—B	386—B	

CHAPTER 8—THE SKIN

Diagrams

389—F	391—A	393—C	394—D
390—E	392—B		

Multiple choice

395—B	397—B	399—A	401—C
396—D	398—C	400—A	

True/false

402—F	410—T	418—T	426—T
403—T	411—T	419—T	427—F

404—F	412—F	420—T	428—T
405—T	413—T	421—F	429—F
406—T	414—F	422—T	430—F
407—T	415—T	423—F	431—T
408—T	416—F	424—T	432—T
409—F	417—T	425—T	433—F

CHAPTER 9—THE URINARY SYSTEM

Diagrams

434—B	439—D	444—A	449—B
435—A	440—D	445—B	450—D
436—F	441—E	446—F	451—E
437—C	442—C	447—A	
438—E	443—F	448—C	

Multiple choice

452—C	454—A	456—D	458—A
453—B	455—C	457—B	

True/false

459—T	463—F	467—F	471—T
460—T	464—T	468—F	472—F
461—F	465—F	469—T	473—T
462—F	466—T	470—T	474—F

Matching items

475—D	476—B	477—E

CHAPTER 10—THE NERVOUS SYSTEM

Diagrams

478—B	488—K	498—D	508—B
479—D	489—A	499—C	509—E
480—A	490—C	500—F	510—C
481—C	491—E	501—H	511—A
482—B	492—J	502—E	512—D
483—D	493—L	503—C	513—B
484—F	494—A	504—D	514—B
485—H	495—I	505—G	515—D
486—G	496—G	506—F	516—C
487—I	497—B	507—A	517—A

Multiple choice

518—C	520—B	521—C	522—C
519—C			

True/false

523—F	531—T	539—F	547—T
524—T	532—F	540—T	548—F
525—F	533—F	541—F	549—F
526—F	534—T	542—F	550—T
527—T	535—T	543—F	551—F
528—F	536—F	544—T	552—T
529—F	537—T	545—T	553—F
530—T	538—F	546—F	554—T

Matching items

555—C	560—C	565—D	570—B
556—D	561—B	566—C	571—D
557—B	562—D	567—D	572—A
558—E	563—A	568—E	
559—A	564—B	569—C	

CHAPTER 11—THE SPECIAL SENSES

Diagrams

573—L	579—E	584—H	589—H
574—I	580—G	585—A	590—C
575—J	581—D	586—I	591—E
576—A	582—C	587—G	592—F
577—K	583—F	588—D	593—B
578—B			

Multiple choice

594—C	595—D	596—B	597—D

True/false

598—T	607—T	616—F	625—T
599—F	608—T	617—T	626—F
600—F	609—F	618—T	627—T
601—T	610—T	619—F	628—T
602—T	611—F	620—T	629—F
603—F	612—T	621—F	630—T
604—T	613—F	622—T	631—F
605—T	614—F	623—T	632—F
606—T	615—F	624—F	633—T

Matching items

634—B	638—B	642—A	646—B
635—C	639—A	643—B	647—E
636—D	640—E	644—D	648—A
637—D	641—D	645—C	

CHAPTER 12—THE ENDOCRINE SYSTEM

Multiple choice

649—D	650—B	651—C	652—D

True/false

653—T	661—T	669—F	677—T
654—F	662—T	670—F	678—T
655—T	663—T	671—F	679—F
656—T	664—T	672—T	680—F
657—T	665—F	673—F	681—F
658—F	666—F	674—F	682—F
659—T	667—T	675—F	683—T
660—F	668—T	676—T	684—T

Missing words

685—A	687—E	689—G	690—H
686—C	688—F		

CHAPTER 13—THE REPRODUCTIVE SYSTEM

Diagrams

691—C	699—D	707—A	715—G
692—A	700—A	708—B	716—B
693—F	701—F	709—F	717—E
694—E	702—B	710—C	718—A
695—B	703—C	711—I	719—D
696—G	704—E	712—D	720—C
697—D	705—J	713—G	721—F
698—E	706—H	714—H	

Multiple choice

722—A	724—C	726—B	728—D
723—B	725—C	727—B	

True/false

729—F	736—T	743—F	750—T
730—T	737—T	744—T	751—F
731—T	738—F	745—T	752—T
732—T	739—T	746—T	753—T
733—F	740—F	747—F	754—F
734—T	741—T	748—T	755—T
735—T	742—T	749—T	756—T

Index

Numbers in **bold** refer to figures or tables

T